# Basic Facts About
# DYSLEXIA
## & Other Reading Problems

# Basic Facts About
# DYSLEXIA
## & Other Reading Problems

by Louisa Cook Moats, Ed.D.,
& Karen E. Dakin, M.Ed.

The International Dyslexia Association
Baltimore, Maryland

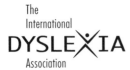

The
International
**DYSLEXIA**
Association

*Promoting literacy through research, education, and advocacy.*™
Founded in Memory of Dr. Samuel T. Orton

The membership of the International Dyslexia Association (IDA) promotes understanding and support of individuals with dyslexia and other learning problems. The headquarters office in Baltimore, Maryland, provides information and referral services to thousands of people every year. For more information on IDA and membership, contact

**The International Dyslexia Association**
40 York Road, 4ᵗʰ Floor
Baltimore, MD 21204-5202
Telephone: (410) 296-0232
(800) ABC-D123
Fax: (410) 321-5069
www.interdys.org

Copyright © 2008 The International Dyslexia Association
All rights reserved
Composition by Type Shoppe II Productions, Ltd.
Printed in the United States of America by Versa Press, Inc., East Peroria, Illinois.

The individuals and situations described in this book are based on the authors' experiences. In all instances, names have been changed; in some instances, identifying details have also been altered to further protect confidentiality.

The description of the partnership between Newgrange Education Center of Princeton, New Jersey, and the Trenton, New Jersey public schools featured in Chapter 6 was graciously provided by Gordon Sherman, Ph.D., Executive Director of the Newgrange School and Educational Outreach Center in New Jersey.

**Library of Congress Cataloging-in-Publication Data**
Moats, Louisa Cook.
  Basic facts about dyslexia & other reading problems / by Louisa Cook Moats and Karen E. Dakin.
      p. cm.
  Includes bibliographical references and index.
  ISBN-13: 978-0-89214-064-0
  ISBN-10: 0-89214-064-X
  1. Dyslexia. 2. Dyslexic children—Education. 3. Reading disability. 4. Learning disabled children. I. Dakin, Karen. II. International Dyslexia Association. III. Title. IV. Title: Basic facts about dyslexia and other reading problems.
  LB1050.5.M597 2007
  371.91'44—dc22

                                                                    2007033664

# Contents

# About the Authors

**Louisa Cook Moats, Ed.D.,** Dr. Moats has been a teacher, psychologist, researcher, graduate school faculty member, and author of many influential scientific journal articles, books, and policy papers on the topics of reading, spelling, language, and teacher preparation. She began her professional career as a neuropsychology technician and teacher of students with learning disabilities. She earned her master's degree at Peabody College of Vanderbilt and her doctorate in Reading and Human Development from the Harvard Graduate School of Education.

Dr. Moats recently spent four years as site director of the NICHD Early Interventions Project in Washington, DC. This longitudinal, large-scale project was conducted through the University of Texas, Houston under the direction of Barbara Foorman, Ph.D. It investigated the causes and remedies for reading failure in high-poverty urban schools. Dr. Moats spent the previous fifteen years in private practice as a licensed psychologist in Vermont, specializing in evaluation and consultation with individuals of all ages who experienced learning problems in reading and language.

Dr. Moats is currently focusing on the improvement of teacher preparation and professional development through her LETRS program (Language Essentials for Teachers of Reading and Spelling). She serves on the National Board of the International Dyslexia Association.

**Karen E. Dakin, M.Ed.,** has been a classroom teacher, reading specialist, resource room teacher, and since 1999, the Director of the Center for Academic Potential at Hathaway Brown School, a large private girls' school in Shaker Heights, Ohio, that serves over 800 girls from pre-school to grade twelve. In this capacity, Ms. Dakin oversees the learning intervention school wide and helps to implement an effective early literacy intervention program. Prior to coming to Hathaway Brown School, Ms. Dakin was the Co-Director of the Learning Assessment Clinic at the Cleveland Clinic Foundation, Cleveland, Ohio, where for 11 years she carried out the educational testing and wrote the summary report for each of the students going through the team's multidisciplinary assessment. Ms. Dakin has also been the Director of her own educational therapy clinic serving children, adolescents, and adults with dyslexia. Ms. Dakin holds a master's degree from Rutgers University and is a certified reading specialist. She has been actively involved with the International Dyslexia Association for almost 30 years and currently serves on its Board of Directors as Vice President.

# Acknowledgments

The authors would like to thank Malt Joshi, Jeff Gilger, and Gordon Sherman for providing detailed editing of earlier versions of the manuscript, and Sandi Soper and Billie Calvery for their helpful reviews. Most of all, we are grateful to Elaine Niefeld and Denise Douce at the IDA office for their publishing expertise, tact, editorial insights, and diligence in bringing this publication to life.

*To our dyslexic students who have taught us so much and to the dedicated teachers everywhere who are devoted to teaching these students how to read.*

# 1

# WHAT IS DYSLEXIA?

*Dyslexia* literally means *difficulty* (dys) with *words* (lex). The term was originally coined and used by medical doctors in the late 1800s. Physicians were the first professionals to develop a scientific interest in why some children had unusual or unexpected difficulty learning to read. Since then, many other professionals have joined physicians in conducting and publishing thousands of studies addressing questions, such as the following:

- How does a good reader read?

- How do students learn to read?

- Why do some students fail to learn easily?

- What is the relationship between language and reading?

- How can we be most helpful to students with problems?

The results of so many studies are helpful for understanding dyslexia, but they can also be confusing. What seems like a problem with a straight-forward definition is called many different things. Developmental reading disorder, developmental reading disability, specific reading disability, specific language disability, intrinsic reading difficulty, and biologically based reading difficulty are just some of the terms used by psychologists, psychiatrists, researchers, reading specialists, and teachers. To further complicate matters, not everyone would define these terms the same way. Consequently, it makes sense to clarify terminology and definitions, even when one professional is talking to another.

## WHY DEFINE DYSLEXIA?

The terms *dyslexia* and *dyslexic* continue to spark controversy. In fact, some school administrators, teachers, parents, and expert professionals refuse to use them. They believe that using the terms *dyslexia* and *dyslexic* leads to misunderstandings about students and their educational needs. On the other hand, some states, such as Texas and Louisiana, test and determine eligibility for teaching services based on a classification of *dyslexia*. Opinions also differ regarding the range of difficulty encompassed by the terms. Some professionals use the term *dyslexic* for individuals with any kind of reading, writing, or language problem. For others, *dyslexic* refers only to students who have specific language-based learning disabilities and who need special, expert instruction to progress in school.

Unfortunately, this controversy can delay or prevent the delivery of services, whereas a formal working definition gives everyone involved a place to begin. It helps *educators* communicate more effectively with each other and with students and their families about the students' learning problems and their educational needs. *Parents* need a definition to help them understand why their child is struggling with learning, and what they can do to help. *Researchers* need the consistent wording or terminology of a definition so other researchers can understand and confirm their findings. The *public*, including *dyslexic adults*, need trustworthy and up-to-date information about dyslexia so that they can pursue the most helpful instruction and accommodations. *Television, newspaper*, and *magazine reporters* need to know what *dyslexia* is to write accurate and informative coverage of the topic.

## A FORMAL DEFINITION

In 2002, experts in reading research and related fields reflected upon the findings of thousands of scientific studies to write a standard definition. Their definition, as approved by the International Dyslexia Association and the Director of Reading Research at the National Institute of Child Health and Human Development, is as follows:

> Dyslexia is a specific learning disability that is neurobiological in origin. It is characterized by difficulties with accurate and/or fluent word recognition and by poor spelling and decoding abilities. These difficulties typically result from a deficit in the phonological component of language that is often unexpected in relation to other cognitive abilities and the provision of effective classroom instruction. Secondary consequences may include problems in reading comprehension and reduced reading experience that can

impede growth of vocabulary and background knowledge. (Lyon, Shaywitz, & Shaywitz, 2003, p. 2)

A more detailed explanation of the key pieces of this definition follows:

- **Specific learning disability** is an impairment of
  learning ability that may affect one or more academic areas, but not others, and that exists in spite
  of adequate intelligence and opportunity to learn.
  For example, a person may be good at math or mechanical problem solving but poor at reading. *Specific
  learning disability* is also defined in special education
  laws and policies, often in different ways by different
  states.

- **Neurobiological in origin** means that the person's
  reading, language, or writing problems arose from
  factors within that individual that have a basis in
  "wired in" aptitudes for language learning and reading. However, the person's environment and experiences in life also determine how well he or she
  learns.

- **Accurate and fluent word recognition** is the person's ability to read single printed words accurately
  and quickly and to read aloud with sufficient speed to
  support understanding.

- **Spelling and decoding abilities** refers to the person's ability to spell accurately and to read unknown
  words by using phonics or letter-sound correspondences and by recognizing syllable patterns and other
  chunks of longer words.

- **A deficit in the phonological component of language** is difficulty pronouncing, remembering, or thinking about the individual speech sounds that make up words.

- **That is often unexpected** means that in spite of typical classroom instruction, adequate intelligence, and opportunity to learn, the person struggles with reading and/or writing more than other students at the same grade, age, or ability level.

- **Secondary consequences** means that students with dyslexia, because they cannot and do not read very much and are not "wired" to learn language easily, often have related problems learning the meanings of words and comprehending academic language as they progress through the grades.

## THE TRUTH ABOUT DYSLEXIA

Even with a standard, working definition, many people remain confused about aspects of dyslexia. The following list addresses some of the questions and misunderstandings on the topic:

- Dyslexia is not primarily a *visual* problem; it is a *language*-based problem.

- Dyslexia does not mean seeing things backwards and is not necessarily indicated by reversals of letters or words.

- Dyslexia or reading disability occurs in people of all levels of intelligence, not just the intellectually gifted.

- Dyslexia is not caused by lack of motivation or interest in reading. Lack of motivation to read and write may be a consequence of dyslexia because reading is very taxing and difficult for a dyslexic individual.

- Dyslexia is not only a problem in families who do not read frequently and together; it can occur in any family.

- Boys and girls are affected by dyslexia, with boys affected somewhat more than girls, but not overwhelmingly so.

## HOW MANY PEOPLE HAVE DYSLEXIA?

Reading ability is distributed according to the normal curve, like height and weight (see Figure 1). Researchers use an arbitrary cutoff point to determine who is classified as dyslexic. In its most severe forms, it is a learning disability and a handicapping condition. In its most mild forms, it may be a source of puzzlement, embarrassment, frustration, irritation, curiosity, and humor. Some dyslexic individuals even like to describe their dyslexia as a "gift" because they believe it coexists with novel and creative problem-solving skills.

No one has statistics on how many people have mild forms of dyslexia, but such problems are very common. Mild

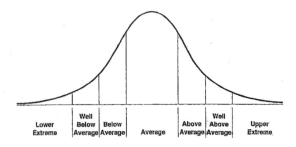

**Figure 1.**   A normal curve showing how reading ability is distributed among the population.

problems with spelling, word pronunciation, phonic decoding, foreign language learning, and language use are ubiquitous or very, very common, even in prominent public figures. In such cases, the term is used to describe a relative weakness in the person's overall profile of abilities. The use of the term does not mean that the person has a handicapping condition that would have qualified him or her for special education services in school. It does convey, however, that the problem may not have yielded to informed instruction, and that it remains an intrinsic and life-long condition.

# 2

# DYSLEXIA

## Manifestations from Preschool to Adulthood

Although it is helpful to agree upon a definition, such as the one in Chapter 1, it is more important to remember that no two dyslexic individuals are exactly alike, and that the manifestations of dyslexia change over time. Experts agree on the core difficulties that characterize a biologically based reading disability, but the following aspects of the disorder vary considerably from one individual to the next:

- Severity of the problem
- Duration of the problem
- Responsiveness of the problem to treatment or remediation
- Relative difficulty a person has with related aspects of reading, spelling, writing, math, or language learning

- Coexisting conditions, or existence of other types of problems with dyslexia, such as anxiety, attention, or word retrieval difficulties

- Coexisting strengths, or areas of talent and interest that enable a person to do well in life, such as visual-spatial, athletic, or intellectual gifts

Keeping these variations in mind, it is still useful to know what is typical at various stages of development to identify a problem and provide help when necessary. The following descriptions of typical manifestations at each age are illustrated with the experiences of children the authors have known. These examples are given as a guide to understanding dyslexia, with the caution that any given individual might vary from what is typical.

## PRESCHOOL: GETTING READY TO READ

Signs of future reading difficulties often emerge before a child goes to school. If a child is late learning to talk, preferring nonverbal gestures and facial expressions over words when communicating with caregivers, the child is at risk for later reading and language difficulties. Such children acquire vocabulary very slowly at a time when more typically developing children are learning several new word meanings every day.

Dyslexic children at this age may also mix up the pronunciations of words much more or for a longer period of time than other children, for example, saying "aminal" for *animal*, "spusgetti" for *spaghetti*, or "emeny" for *enemy*, even after multiple corrections. They may have persistent trouble with difficult speech sounds such as /th/, /r/, /l/, and /w/.

The preschool child who is at risk for dyslexia may not enjoy looking at or following the print when books are read aloud. David, for example, is a five-year-old in pre-kindergarten who struggles to remember the letters in his name. He confuses the names of letters and numbers, sometimes identifying a letter as a number or vice versa. Many children with dyslexia at this age will seem impatient when read to or disinterested in books, preferring other kinds of play. David does not enjoy word play, such as making rhymes, repeating traditional nursery rhymes, saying strings of words with the same beginning sound, or making up silly names for people. For children such as David, letter names and shapes may be hard to remember even if family members or preschool teachers encourage games such as matching and naming letter shapes.

Unlike David, some children in prekindergarten readily learn to identify and write the letters of the alphabet and to write their names, but oral communication that involves comprehending questions, directions, and explanations or responding appropriately may be an obvious challenge. For example, a child might be confused about the meaning of the words *who, what, where,* and *when*. When her mother asks, "Where is your doll?" the child answers, "I like my doll." Or, if asked about the color of her backpack, she might say, "I wear my backpack to school."

Other preschool children at risk for dyslexia may do fine with listening, speaking, and verbal comprehension. Their problems are confined to print-related activities that do not become apparent until kindergarten or first grade.

## Screening and Early Identification in Preschool

Preschool children whose language development is seriously delayed are at very high risk for reading difficulties in kindergarten and first grade, even if they receive extra help developing oral language skills before kindergarten. Carol, for example, was identified in preschool as needing language therapy to improve her listening comprehension and oral expression skills; she had particular difficulty with word retrieval. After two years of therapy, she continued to struggle with early literacy tasks, such as rhyming and understanding that letters represent sounds.

Language comprehension and expression problems are often associated with later reading problems; that is one reason why all preschool children's language development should be screened at ages 3 and 4, and language therapy programs begun early if problems are detected. Fortunately, educators now have well-researched screening instruments that assist in the identification of potentially dyslexic children very early, before they fail. Carol, for example, benefited greatly from the combination of very early language help and additional small group, structured language work once she was in school.

## KINDERGARTEN AND FIRST GRADE: BEGINNING TO READ

By kindergarten, most children begin the process of learning the alphabet to read and write. For some, it happens quickly and with relatively little effort. For others, it is a gradual process. For the kindergarten child with a predisposition for dyslexia, it can be particularly slow. For this child, the mystery of letter names and sounds may remain just that, a mystery. Some children navigate the social learning part of kindergarten very well, but begin to realize by mid-kindergarten that they are not catching on to letters and sounds as quickly as their peers. Certainly, by the first few weeks of first grade, children can tell if they are lagging behind. Even though they may not realize or know how to tell an adult that they are worried about reading, they may begin to show frustration and anxiety, and in some cases, avoid school altogether.

A primary literacy goal for a kindergarten child is to develop *phonemic awareness*: the ability to identify and manipulate the individual speech sounds in spoken words. A phoneme is the smallest unit of speech in our language, a sound such as the /f/, /l/, /a/, or /sh/ in *flash*. When phonemic awareness is achieved, the child can then go on to decode words by letter-sounds, to recognize whole words, and to spell.

The child who has difficulty detecting and creating rhyme will usually have difficulty acquiring phonemic awareness. This child may have memorized how to read or spell *cat*, but have no understanding of how to read or spell *fat*. He or she does not understand that the letters in the alphabet represent speech sounds in words. Educators often describe this problem as lack of understanding of the *alphabetic principle*—that letters represent phonemes or speech sounds.

Other early signs of reading difficulty include trouble with the following learning activities:

- Remembering the names of letters and recalling them quickly
- Recalling the sounds that the letters represent

- Learning to recognize common words (family names; names on signs or objects, such as cereal boxes; or the most common words used in writing) by sight, or automatically

- Spelling the sounds of words in a plausible way so the words can be recognized by the reader

It is important, though, to keep in mind that a child can have these oral and written language learning problems and, at the same time, show talents, interests, and abilities in many other areas that have nothing to do with reading. The child may therefore be very puzzling to him or herself and to family members.

### Screening in Kindergarten and First Grade

If the reading problem is identified by the end of first grade, and the child is taught the direct connection between letters and sounds, he or she should make good progress. Otherwise, the dyslexic student will move on to second or third grade with certain critical reading and writing behaviors that set them apart from their peers. Unfortunately, for this student and many others, the wonderful world of reading will remain a mystery.

## SECOND AND THIRD GRADE

After 2 or 3 years of schooling, dyslexic children may have learned some skills, but they typically demonstrate continuing difficulties with reading, spelling, and writing. If language and reading difficulties have not been fully remediated by second and third grade, a student with dyslexia will almost always have three predictable, observable problems:

- Inability to recognize important and common words by sight, or instantly, without having to laboriously sound them out

- Faltering during the sounding out or letter-sound association (decoding) process, and recalling the wrong sounds for the letters and letter patterns

- Poor spelling, with speech sounds omitted (e.g., the word *after* spelled *afr*), wrong letters for sounds used (e.g., the word *sing* spelled *san*), and poor recall for even frequently used "little" words, such as *when, went, they, their, been, to, does, said,* and *what*

When children with reading disabilities are reading a passage aloud, they may read word by word and without expression because they are using all their available attention to determine the meaning of each individual word. Reading feels—to them and to the listener—like very hard work. Their reading is *dysfluent,* meaning that it is too slow and lacks appropriate expression, and it is marked by many decoding or word recognition errors. Typically, the child tries to guess at unknown words on the basis of pictures, the story theme, or one or two letters in the word, instead of using knowledge of phonics to decode the whole word from left to right.

Spelling, handwriting, and written composition are almost always the latest developing skills for the dyslexic student, and at this age, many children do everything they can to avoid writing. Jason, for example, struggles with learning to write his letters. He is not sure where to place his pencil to start each letter, and, therefore, does not have a kinesthetic pattern, or familiar way to move his hand, to correctly form each letter. He reverses the letters *b* and *d*, and also *c, g,* and *z.* Spelling is a big problem for Jason.

Writing is the most demanding of all the language skills we learn in school; it requires a mental and physical juggling act of unparalleled complexity that is challenging for many students. However, this is even truer for dyslexic students. They may spend a tremendous amount of time with little to show for their efforts and have inordinate difficulty with the symbol-usage parts of writing (spelling, punctuation, letter formation, and spacing). Jason studies nightly to memorize the spelling words for the week, and he often achieves a reasonable grade on his test, sometimes even a perfect score. However, in his mind, spelling words are not organized around a particular pattern, so he forgets how to spell those same words a week later. So many tasks, including remembering which way the pencil goes, spelling the most common words, and organizing thoughts into sentences and paragraphs, can be daunting for the dyslexic student.

Many other problems may coexist with these core symptoms, such as avoidance of reading and writing assignments, difficulty producing homework within a reasonable time frame, poor memory for verbal information, inattention to the teacher's voice when distractions are present, and language comprehension problems. In Jason's case, he resorts to short, simple words in his writing even though he readily uses more interesting vocabulary to tell stories. As the writing demands increase, so do Jason's stomachaches.

Fortunately, students have other strengths, such as artistic, athletic, mechanical, social, mathematical, or scientific abilities. Jason, for example, has excellent oral language skills. By recognizing and encouraging Jason's strengths early and frequently, he might have fewer stomachaches as he experiences success in other areas, such as debate or drama.

## Transition to Reading to Learn

By the end of third grade, students are expected to know how to read. For most students, the critical transition from third grade to fourth is from learning to read to reading to learn. This transition can be overwhelming for the dyslexic student. By the fourth grade, Bill was reading at only a mid-second-grade level, even though he received help to address his difficulty with similar sounding words. His lingering phonological (speech sound awareness) problems affected his ability in both oral language comprehension and reading comprehension. Comprehension becomes more critical in these transitional grades as students are expected to gain new knowledge of challenging content from their reading assignments, both in class and on their own. In a typical fourth-grade classroom, teachers no longer teach children to read, with the possible exception of teaching comprehension strategies and skills.

Another difficulty for dyslexic students in the intermediate grades is the change in the nature of the reading. More of the reading is nonfiction, and the strategies that helped the dyslexic reader in second grade may no longer work. He or she may be good in math concepts and problem solving, but misread the directions or word problems. Context is not as reliable with science and social studies reading; vocabulary and pictures are not as plentiful or helpful. The dyslexic child frequently struggles to keep up, often taking unfinished class work home in addition to the regular homework. Parents spend hours reading the material to their child and writing the answers to save time. This dependency on others takes its toll on the child's self-esteem and feeling of competence.

## INTERMEDIATE GRADES, FOURTH TO SIXTH

The dyslexic student in the intermediate grades may have key symptoms of dyslexia, even if he or she has received expert instruction. The core difficulty, reading printed words accurately and fluently, remains, even though the child may be making good progress learning to decode or decipher unknown words. On the surface, the child's problem is reflected on timed oral reading tests that ask the student to read a passage aloud for 1 minute. Referred to as oral reading fluency (ORF), these short, timed tests are key indicators of overall reading proficiency. Difficulty with ORF is most often caused by underlying, residual problems with recognizing sight words and matching letters to speech sounds.

Several other indicators are critical for distinguishing the dyslexic child from children who simply lack reading practice:

- The dyslexic child will typically do poorly when asked to read lists of single, common words that are taken out of the context of a paragraph. When words are put into lists, the child can no longer depend on the context of the story or sentence to guess them.

- The child will usually do even more poorly on a test of reading nonsense words. Reading nonsense words, such as *pem*, *loit*, and *thwadge*, requires the use of letter-sound correspondences or phonic patterns, a skill that is difficult for students with dyslexia.

- The child's spelling is still poor.
- The child may have trouble with a comprehension question on a reading test, but often does much better when comprehension is measured through tests that do not require reading.

## Screening and Intervention in the Intermediate Grades

If left untreated or unrecognized, the reading and writing problems of the dyslexic student will continue through middle school and can become even more entrenched. Students with dyslexia do not teach themselves to read and write just because they are surrounded by print every day. Rather, they become better at getting along without reading and writing.

By the end of the intermediate grades, if the remedial instruction is not strong enough, if it was started very late, or if the teacher is not aware of or sensitive to the nature of the child's difficulty, the dyslexic child in the regular classroom may resort to either maladaptive or constructive coping strategies. Maladaptive coping strategies include avoiding reading and writing at all costs; becoming hostile or resistant to schooling in general; or becoming depressed or antisocial and looking to nonacademic activities for self-esteem or social validation.

More constructive and adaptive coping strategies include relying on other sources for information, including electronic media; obtaining help with note-taking, technology use, and test preparation; learning to advocate for one's own needs; and starting assignments very early. Technology, in particular, is a vital tool for the dyslexic student at this stage. Children who struggle with handwriting can become competent with a keyboard. Some dyslexic students are so adept with their word processing that they can take notes on their laptops as early as fourth grade. They comment that their spelling is much improved on the laptop, even without the support of a spell checker. Other technology allows students to scan their reading assignments into a computer that then reads the words back through a print-to-voice synthesizer. There are also computer programs that provide a pronunciation or definition for any word in a text that the student is reading on the monitor.

As Bill's reading skills improved, he became passionate about the computer. In order to do what he wanted on the computer, he spent considerable time reading as he used the computer. He found that it helped with his writing, too. The computer helped Bill become an organized, self-motivated student before he faced the new challenges of middle and high school.

But a word of caution—although assistive technology can be a great support to the dyslexic learner, it remains imperative that critical reading and writing skills still be taught directly so dyslexic students become competent and bridge the gap between their skills and those of their classmates.

## MIDDLE AND HIGH SCHOOL

The dyslexic student, who might have been able to cope in the intermediate grades with support and remediation, may quickly fall apart in middle and high school. Middle and high school programs are organized in such a way that students have a different teacher for each subject, and the entire day requires multiple physical and intellectual transitions and adjustments. The volume of work and the amount of self-direction required, as well as the demands on time and space management, may all exceed the student's coping skills.

By middle school, in addition to the core language, reading, and writing problems with which the student began, the student's most apparent needs shift to note-taking skills, notebook organization, schedule compliance and time management, independent study habits, homework completion, and strategies for dealing with a slow reading rate.

Delivery of remedial instruction also becomes more and more difficult as students progress to higher grade levels. Middle and high schools seldom give credit for remedial reading and writing courses, although the students may need up to 2 hours of instruction daily to gain ground on their peers. School counselors and specialists tend to focus on academic accommodations for dyslexic students, such as extra time on tests, shortened assignments, help with word processing or note taking, recorded texts, and so forth. These services are important and necessary, but specialized academic skill instruction is also needed to continue any gains made previously, and accommodations cannot substitute for reading and writing instruction. Students at this level may know that they are not progressing in fundamental academic skills, even though they may be given passing grades, and this experience may further alienate and frustrate them.

Another area of potential concern for the high school student with dyslexia is high stakes testing. Grace, a high school junior, was referred for psychoeducational testing by her math tutor. She was an A/B student in high school, but a slow reader. Her tutor was concerned that Grace's performance on important college admission tests would not reflect her true understanding of the material being tested, whether on math or verbal tests. Many high school students, like Grace, need accommodations on high stakes testing such as state proficiency tests and testing for the college admission process.

Grace's psychoeducational assessment revealed that she was a gifted dyslexic whose phonological skills and rapid naming skills were still very weak, even though she was quite a competent reader. In addition to working with an educational specialist skilled in remediating dyslexia with the goal of becoming a more efficient reader and writer, Grace also began receiving accommodations in school, primarily extended time on assignments and tests. The additional time made a huge difference for her on the college admission testing, and she achieved a 4.0 academic average her senior year of high school.

## Accommodations for High Stakes Testing

When requesting accommodations for high stakes testing, it is important to include specifics about the student's disability. Grace was initially turned down by college testing services for the accommodation of extended time, but she submitted a letter of appeal stating that her phonological skills were well below average and she was inordinately slow in some basic processes underlying reading, such as rapid symbol naming. Once the College Board reviewed the specifics of the appeal, they granted the accommodation. The same definition of dyslexia given in Chapter 1 was referenced in the appeal letter that acknowledged Grace's dyslexia and her need for extended time.

## COLLEGE AND ADULTHOOD

Occasionally, a person may not be diagnosed as dyslexic until college or professional school, when the demands of reading and writing become so great that they jeopardize the individual's success in his or her chosen field. Jeff sought help when, as a surgery resident in his final year, he was having considerable difficulty keeping up with his reading. He was also distressed by the frequent rejections he received from publishers because his writing required so much revision. Looking back, Jeff realized that he had avoided the problem throughout college. Reading synopses of books and avoiding classes with a lot of required reading had gotten Jeff through college—but now his career was at stake.

Dyslexic individuals who succeed in college or postsecondary education usually need accommodations for a slow reading rate, note-taking difficulties, and problems with written composition. Those accommodations may include extra time on tests and assignments, proofreading help, services of a volunteer note-taker for lecture classes, availability of detailed course outlines to support studying, and a quiet space for test taking to reduce distractions. Many seek extra support from college academic services and carefully choose courses wisely that are a good match for their strengths. They may also request alternatives to learning a foreign language, not because they cannot learn another language, but because the circumstances and conditions of college classroom instruction may not be manageable. For example, many foreign language courses in college emphasize rapid auditory-verbal drills that are difficult for dyslexic students.

Every field, from law to medicine to teaching, has professionals who are dyslexic. Professors of philosophy and other academic areas at highly selective colleges have succeeded in college and graduate school because their field requires very slow, thoughtful reading, and they can hire proofreaders to correct their spelling and grammar. Many others, including lawyers, actors, writers, painters, business executives, and members of every other profession are dyslexic. Many overcame their worst problems with reading and writing by following a passionate interest in a topic area or field of study that propelled them through the worst periods of frustration. This passion gave them the motivation to persist during demanding and uncomfortable reading and writing tasks. A strong interest, hard work, and perseverance have carried many dyslexic adults through the toughest period of their lives—school!—and enabled them to succeed in every possible walk of life.

# 3

# HOW COMMON
# IS THE PROBLEM?

## READING DIFFICULTY IS COMMON

Researchers agree that difficulty with reading is a widespread problem. On the measure used across most of the United States, the National Assessment of Educational Progress (NAEP), about 38% of all fourth grade students are described as having "below basic" reading skills. Students such as these, who are at or below the 40th percentile for their age group (those who do not read as well as 60% of their peers), are at some risk for failing the high-stakes, year-end achievement tests used by most states. Those with milder problems (those who score between the 20th and 40th percentiles on a screening test) have about a 50% chance of failing an end-of-year reading achievement test. Those who score below the 20th percentile on a screening test of basic reading skill are very likely to fail end-of-year, state-administered tests. Children in the bottom 20% are clearly "below grade level" in reading and are unlikely to improve their relative standing without expert, intensive instruction.

Another way to state these facts is that 40% of the population is likely to have academic achievement problems related to inadequate reading skills. In minority and high poverty schools, that figure is as high as 70–80%. Nationwide, 20% of the elementary school population is clearly struggling with reading, is at clear risk for academic failure, and is in need of remedial intervention or specialized instruction; that is, 1 child in 5, or at least 4 children per an average classroom of 20 children.

## ADULT ILLITERACY

The United States Department of Education also keeps statistics on adult literacy. The most recent National Assessment of Adult Literacy (2003), reported by the National Center for Education Statistics, showed that 5% of all adults are "non-literate," about the same proportion as children in education research studies who have chronic, severe, reading disabilities. These adults cannot read at all. Another 21–23% of adults can recognize some words but function at the lowest level of reading, often described as *functional illiteracy*. In other words, we can safely say that 20–25% of the adult population can only read at the lowest level or not at all. Of this 20–25% of non-literate and non-reading adults, only about 25% are immigrants whose command of English is limited; 62% dropped out of high school, suggesting that their problems were chronic and began early in school; and about 44% live below the poverty level. Only about

26% of the non-literate and non-reading adults have documented physical, intellectual, or mental health disabilities. So, how can we explain the reading difficulties of the majority of adult poor readers?

## DYSLEXIA IS ONE EXPLANATION FOR THE PROBLEM

Some individuals, even if they receive good instruction and are motivated to learn, have trouble learning to read. Research suggests that there are three major reasons why. First, they may not know how to read and spell words accurately because they have trouble associating sounds with letters and the letter patterns in words. This is the core problem for approximately 70–80% of students with poor reading skills. Second, some individuals cannot read words or text fast enough to comprehend what they are reading. They can read words accurately, but they have trouble developing *automaticity* in word recognition, the instant recognition of printed words. It is estimated that about 10–15% of the students with reading difficulties have this problem. Third, some students never developed the reasoning ability, background knowledge, or language skills to make sense of what they read. They can read words accurately and quickly, but they have trouble connecting meaning to the decoded words. Sometimes, the terms *hyperlexic* or *word caller* are used for that third group, which comprises about 10–15% of students with reading disabilities.

Not everyone agrees that all of these difficulties are attributable to dyslexia. According to the definition in Chapter 1, dyslexia is a specific learning disability that is neurobiological in origin. It is unexpected, given the individual's opportunities to learn, and a problem that most often begins with weakness in the phonological (speech sound) aspects of language processing. In other words, students in the first group, those who early in their development have trouble developing speech sound awareness and memory for the speech sounds that alphabetic symbols represent, are dyslexic. But some researchers use the term *dyslexic* to apply broadly to children in all three groups, pointing out that dyslexia is very common and present in virtually every classroom.

Testing has not resolved this debate. The NAEP test requires students to read passages silently and answer multiple-choice questions; it does not measure reading rate or the ability to recognize single words out of the context of a passage. Therefore, it is not possible to know from this assessment how many of these students who are "below basic" have prominent difficulties recognizing the words, as would be the case with dyslexia. A separate study of the NAEP students' oral reading fluency (ORF) was conducted in the last few years, however, and those students whose reading rates were slow were highly likely to be among those who did poorly on the reading comprehension passages. Slow reading is itself an indicator of poor word recognition, but other factors, such as weak vocabulary knowledge may contribute to the overall problem, for example, as is the case for students in the third group who lack background knowledge. Furthermore, the types of reading difficulty rarely present themselves in a clear-cut way. It is much more common that reading problems are caused by a mix of factors that can be difficult or impossible to sort out, even with extensive and expensive batteries of diagnostic tests.

Medical science has also failed to resolve the debate. There is no genetic or neurological test that conclusively determines the biological underpinnings that predispose a child toward reading disability. That is to say, it cannot be specified with certainty, for a given individual, how much of the problem experienced is neurobiological in origin, and how much is environmentally or experientially caused. It can only be said, on the basis of large-scale scientific research with population groups, that genetic and neurobiological factors determine about half of what goes into learning to read. It can only be inferred that the student who readily responds to instruction has an experience-based problem, and the student who responds slowly to good instruction can blame his or her "wiring" or neurobiological predisposition. We usually reserve the term *dyslexic* for children whose reading, spelling, and language difficulties persist even when they receive excellent instruction.

## THE ROLE OF RESPONSE TO INSTRUCTION

No matter what the cause or type of reading problem, students in the bottom 20% in basic reading skill are likely to be there for the duration of schooling unless something is done to help them overcome their problem. They do not spontaneously learn to read, and very few are late bloomers when it comes to reading. However, if the reading difficulties experienced by these children are identified early, and expert remediation is provided, most of them can be brought up into the average range in basic reading skill.

## WHAT DO THE STATISTICS TELL US?

The statistics in this chapter do not provide all the answers, but they do alert us to the prevalence and seriousness of reading problems as summarized below:

- At least one fifth, or 20% of the population are predisposed to have significant difficulty with reading, and another 20% are at some risk and need some help to get on track and stay on track.

- Percentages of children at risk are much higher in high poverty, language-minority populations who attend ineffective schools.

- The causes for reading difficulty may be neurobiological, experiential, instructional, or a combination of these factors.

- At present, there is no genetic or neurological test to diagnose or predict whose problems are primarily neurobiological.

- About three quarters of the children who show primary difficulties with basic reading skill early in reading development can be helped to overcome those difficulties to a large extent.

- About 5% of the population will have enduring, severe reading disabilities that are very difficult to treat given our current knowledge.

# 4

# IDENTIFYING THE CHILD AT RISK

Early identification and intervention with students who show the warning signs of dyslexia are critically important for better outcomes later on. Scientists have identified the specific skill weaknesses that predict later reading difficulties, making early testing, identification, and remediation possible. For most children, problems can be remediated with programs at the kindergarten and first-grade levels that take about 30–45 minutes per day.

## WHAT ARE THE CRITICAL SKILLS FOR READING?

To become successful readers, children must master the following critical skills:

- Phonological awareness
- Automatic and accurate letter naming
- Letter-sound association
- Word reading accuracy and fluency
- Passage reading fluency and comprehension

A detailed description of each of these skills follows, along with methods for early identification and testing for reading difficulties.

## Phonological Awareness

Reading requires the ability to accurately and rapidly recognize and name single words in print. It is this basic skill that most differentiates the dyslexic student from students who do not like to read and those who lack the intellectual ability to read. Word recognition depends on a specific linguistic ability known as *phonological awareness*. Children with dyslexia are typically slow and inaccurate when they try to link written alphabetic symbols with the sounds they represent, and they often make mistakes when they try to blend those sounds together to read a new word. Conversely, when they try to spell, they have trouble identifying the separate sounds in words and recalling the letters that spell them. They may have a poor sense of how words are put together at both the sound and symbol levels. A child may know how to spell the word *cat* and know the sound for *f*, but have no understanding of how to spell the word *fat*. For example, a child in kindergarten with dyslexia may be able to name all letters correctly and produce the single sounds associated with many of the letters, but when asked to spell a simple two- or three-sound word, such as *him*, the child writes "mpe."

The phonological awareness problem of dyslexic students does not necessarily interfere with their ability to listen for the meanings of language or to pronounce words, although some children do have trouble with enunciation of some sounds and some sound sequences, and some children confuse vocabulary words that sound similar, such as *half* and *have*, and *catch* and *cash*. The central problem that interferes with reading is an inability to separate mentally the speech sounds within spoken words. Consciously separating speech sounds in words is an unnatural, acquired skill for those who learn to read and write, because words are spoken as undivided bursts of sound. Awareness of the internal structure of any spoken word is by nature elusive until we are taught, and even then, individuals vary greatly in the ease with which they learn to analyze words. A dyslexic child or novice reader who is asked to say the first sound in the word *dog* might answer, "bow-wow!" because the question itself does not make sense. The whole word *dog is* one sound to the untrained ear. It is only in reading and spelling that awareness of individual speech sounds is required of children, not in ordinary conversation.

Tasks used to assess phonological awareness in young children usually do not use letters. Instead, children are asked to break words apart into component speech sounds to compare and match speech sounds in words or to blend separate speech sounds into a whole word. More advanced tasks involve taking a speech sound away from a word and saying what is left. The following examples are teacher prompts for testing the phonological skill of a young child who has not yet learned to read:

- Move a penny into a box each time you say a sound in the word *lack* (see Figure 1). (The child puts the first penny in the first box while saying the sound /l/, the second penny in the second box while saying the sound /a/, and the third penny in the third box while saying the sound /k/.

- Which word begins with the same sound as *far*?

  star
  fade
  then
  (Answer: *fade*)

- Listen. /z/ /oo/ /m/. What's the word?

  (Answer: *zoom*)

- Say *face*. Now say the last sound first and the first sound last. What's the word?

  (Answer: *safe*)

- Say *small*. Say it again without /s/. What's the word?

  (Answer: *mall*)

How do we know that phonological awareness skills are causally related to growth in reading skill? First, children who are good at these tasks are much more likely than

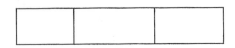

**Figure 1.** Boxes used by the student to indicate each sound in a word.

others to be good readers and spellers. But second, when children are randomly assigned to instructional groups, those who receive instruction in awareness of speech sounds and phonics (use of letter-sound associations to read and spell) are much less likely to be poor readers and much more likely to be good readers than children who do not receive explicit instruction in the speech sounds. Awareness of the separate speech sounds enables children to make a mental map of the correspondences between the letters in printed words and the sounds they represent.

## Automatic and Accurate Letter Naming

A second critical skill that predicts later reading is the ability to recognize and name letters automatically, or without a lot of mental effort. This simple skill, which is easily measured by brief, timed tests of naming letters randomly sequenced in an array, encompasses a number of cognitive or mental skills that are important for reading. First, the

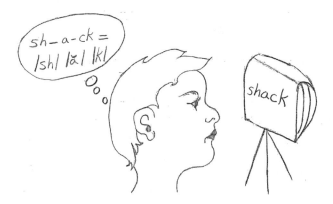

**Figure 2.** A child associates phonemes and graphemes to make a mental map of a word. Drawing by Betsy Denning.

reader must recognize the form of the letter and not confuse it with others—a necessity for associating it with the right speech sound. Second, the reader must recognize written symbols rapidly because this skill is the basis for later automatic recognition of letter sequences that represent *sight words* (i.e., words recognized instantly). Third, letter names are phonological entities composed of speech sounds, some of which are the sounds that the letters represent; for example, the letter *s* has the sound /s/ in the name of the letter. This is true for many letters, such as *b*, *t*, *d*, and *v*, but not for *y*, *h*, and *w*. Thus, children may develop an incorrect generalization that the name for each letter always helps to generate the sound associated with that letter. Letter naming places strong demands on the child's ability to recall the speech sounds that are in the name, in response to seeing a visual symbol. Letter naming tasks measure both phonological (i.e., speech sound) and orthographic (i.e., letter recognition) functions that are critical for beginning reading.

## Letter-Sound Association

A third critical skill that should be directly assessed is the ability to link speech sounds with written symbols. Often referred to as *phonic knowledge,* the matching of speech sounds with letter symbols must be accurate and automatic for a student to decode an unknown word. Otherwise, the student will try to guess at words based on the meaning of the passage or sentence. Tasks whereby children are asked to say the sounds that letters and letter combinations represent are as good at predicting later reading as timed letter naming.

Some children may make the association of the sound to the written symbol, the letter, but still may need a lot of direct instruction and practice to use that knowledge during reading and spelling. For example, a child may have learned the sounds for the letters and letter combinations *a, b, ou,* and *t,* but not know how to read or spell the word *about.* This child may have mastered some knowledge of phonics, but has not received sufficient practice to carry those skills over to real reading. Thus, timed reading of whole words is the next skill that should be assessed.

## Word Reading Accuracy and Fluency

As children become more proficient at the more basic skills already described, *the goal of phonics instruction is to develop automatic or fast recognition of whole words,* or *sight recognition* for fluent, automatic reading. Various well-standardized tests exist for measuring a child's ability to read words in a list. Both the accuracy of word reading and the relative speed with which the child reads the words are important to measure. Some tests include lists of real words and lists of nonsense words for the child to read within a short period. Nonsense word reading is the most stringent test of phonic decoding ability, but real word reading is the skill most closely related to fluent oral reading of meaningful passages. How well a student accurately reads single words in lists usually predicts how well the student will read and comprehend passages.

Sometimes the purpose and role of single word reading is misunderstood. *Sight word recognition* is not achieved by memorizing words on flash cards or by trying to avoid addressing the child's difficulty with phonics. Accurate word reading depends first on understanding the alphabetic code and recognizing the internal details of spoken and written words. Multisensory, structured language teaching, which includes lots of supported practice in accurate and meaningful reading of written words and text, is the most effective path to more fluent reading.

### Passage Reading Fluency and Comprehension

After about the end of first grade, one of the best overall indicators of reading skill is *oral reading fluency* (ORF). Oral reading fluency is the number of words read correctly in 1 minute when a child reads a passage at an appropriate level of difficulty. To check comprehension, the child is also asked to retell what he or she read or to answer questions about the passage. Researchers have collected sufficient data to establish the typical level of oral reading fluency for each grade level.

If a child's oral reading fluency is below the norm for his or her grade level, the reason for that slow or inaccurate oral reading must be established by testing phonemic awareness, automatic and accurate letter naming, letter-sound association skills, and word reading accuracy and fluency. Those students who seem to have all the underlying skills in place but who have specific problems with comprehension will need more extensive testing of vocabulary, listening comprehension, verbal reasoning, attention, and other related skills.

## WHY ARE THE CRITICAL READING SKILLS SO IMPORTANT FOR EARLY IDENTIFICATION AND INTERVENTION?

When young students encounter difficulty with the foundational skills of reading, including phonological awareness, letter naming, the ability to match letter symbols with sounds, or accurate and efficient word recognition, they fall behind their peers right from the beginning. These skills can be taught, but the longer they go untaught, the steeper the hill the student must climb. Even by late kindergarten and early first grade, students who have not mastered basic skills will miss opportunities to practice accurately reading words. Without sufficient word recognition practice, gained through skill instruction and reading, students gain reading fluency more slowly. When students read more slowly, they read less, and they have fewer opportunities to expand their vocabulary and get on with the business of reading for meaning.

A student who has not mastered the alphabetic principle and who does not know the useful phonic correspondences in English will quickly fall behind in terms of the number of words he or she has read. If this "gap" is allowed to develop for too long, it is very difficult to make up the difference in reading experience that, in turn, supports the development of accurate and fluent word recognition. It is possible to "close the gap" in phonological and phonics skills with older children who have reading disabilities, but those individuals typically have enduring problems with reading rate (reading fluency) and consequent problems with vocabulary and comprehension, especially on timed tests.

## HOW CAN WE IDENTIFY STUDENTS AT RISK?

Early screening tests can be powerful predictors of later reading achievement. Simple tasks should be included in any predictive battery of tests designed to locate children

at risk so that intervention can begin early. Experts who
have examined the relative usefulness of specific tasks for
predicting who will develop symptoms have reported the
following findings:

- Timed tests of letter naming or letter-sound associations are the most accurate and powerful single
  predictors of later reading achievement in kindergarten and early first grade.

- Phonemic awareness tasks are useful at the kindergarten and beginning first-grade level, but they tend to
  identify a lot of children as being at risk, when in fact,
  they will not have trouble later (i.e., false positives).
  Children's responses to instruction should be monitored closely so that those who have intrinsic, hard-to-
  remediate problems can be identified early and flagged
  as potentially reading disabled.

- After the middle of first grade, when some instruction
  has been given, better tests involve direct measures of
  decoding and word recognition, the use of phonic
  knowledge to decode simple real and nonsense words.
  Nonsense words that are actually detached syllables,
  such as *tat* (as in *tat*tered), *blem* (as in em*blem*), or *ston*
  (as in a*ston*ish), are used to make sure the child can
  read unfamiliar words. Reading simple real words
  alone may be deceiving because a child may have
  memorized them as sight words and not actually mastered the critical decoding skills.

- As soon as children can read sentences and paragraphs, the best screening measure is oral reading fluency, a timed test that combines reading rate and

accuracy. Oral reading fluency tests should always ask children to respond to comprehension questions. Fluency tests, used with other tests, can help educators find those unusual students who read accurately, but very slowly, and whose fluency problems may constitute a reading handicap.

- The subgroup of children who read accurately but have problems with comprehension are the most difficult to assess because the least is known about them. At a minimum, their understanding of word meanings can be assessed quite easily, and overall language function can be screened by a speech/language therapist.

Once children are receiving reading instruction, their progress should be monitored quite frequently with alternate forms of phonemic awareness, letter naming, phonic decoding, and oral reading fluency tasks. Comprehension should always be taken into account using retelling, summarizing, multiple-choice questions, sentence completion tasks, and other techniques. A child's response to instruction is a critical indicator of the nature and severity of his or her reading difficulty.

# 5

# GENETICS, THE BRAIN, AND DYSLEXIA

---

## ARE PEOPLE BORN WITH DYSLEXIA?

The science of genetics has exploded in the last two decades with improved technologies that have allowed scientists to examine the extent to which many human traits are inherited. Many studies conducted over more than 20 years with several generations of families and with twins raised apart and together, for example, have contributed enormously to our understanding of whether, and how, differences among people in their ability to read are inherited. The not-so-simple answer to the question "Are differences in the ability to read inherited?" is "Yes, in part, but in an indirect and complex way."

Genes do not cause reading disorders directly. There is no one dyslexia gene. Genes give rise to, set the stage for, or give people a tendency toward difficulties or proficiencies with specific kinds of language skills that are necessary for reading and writing. In general, genes provide a predisposition for reading abilities at the high and low end of the ability scale and everywhere in between. In fact, several specific genes have been identified that influence the development and function of the language systems of the brain that are most important for reading.

Thus far, there appear to be a finite number of genes most pertinent for reading skill acquisition, probably less than 10, but more than several. These genes likely interact with each other and the 30,000 or so other genes in humans. If you add environmental effects, you can see how complicated it becomes to determine a person's risk for a reading disability.

Our best estimates suggest that genetics account for about half of the risk for a reading problem. Put another way, genetics account for about half of the variability between people and how they perform on reading and spelling achievement tests. The other half of the equation is probably such factors as methods and length of instruction, the social context for reading, persistence and motivation of individuals, and more. Therefore, a person may have a genetic predisposition for reading difficulty, but with expert instruction early in life, he or she may avoid having a serious reading problem. Unfortunately, it is also possible for a person to have "good genes" for reading, but still suffer setbacks if appropriate instruction is not available.

One way to understand how the genetic inheritance of reading achievement works is to compare it to the genetics of body type and weight control. We tend to inherit a particular body type, a degree of hand-eye coordination, and a certain amount of gross motor skill. For example, some of us seem "born" to be athletes or dancers, while others of us are not so blessed. Nevertheless, if a non-athlete exercises, develops healthy eating habits for weight control, and practices an athletic skill, he or she can become a better athlete. On the other hand, a "born" athlete can fail to capitalize on that genetic gift and become an inactive, overweight, out-of-shape adult!

## HOW DO GENES INFLUENCE READING DEVELOPMENT?

We do not have genes for reading and spelling, per se, but there are genes that influence the development of brain areas responsible for variations in language abilities. Language is a natural and universal human characteristic, while reading is a culturally determined, recently acquired, and unnatural human characteristic. The human brain is not designed to read; learning to read requires the activation of several areas of the brain that are mainly located in the language regions or areas of the brain. For example, awareness of speech sounds in words, memory for letter sequences, memory for word meanings, and other basic processes involved in reading may each be affected by genetics. Brain development in each of several language areas necessary for reading is shaped by genes, although scientists are not yet sure exactly how genes determine brain structure and function.

Genes and the environment work together to influence how we learn. Genes provide a blueprint for neurological development, but many events intervene to determine exactly how those genetic potentials are realized. Overall language abilities are moderately heritable. Again, about half of our skill with language seems to be inherited. This means that if our parents have a gift for language, we are also likely to have an aptitude for or a facility with language. The opposite is also true: if our parents lacked that aptitude or facility, most likely, we will, as well. However, within that general principle, genetic influences on language and reading vary in their effects on behavior. In other words, some children from stimulating and supportive language environments are resistant to language input and instruction. They seem to have traits that are hard wired. Others, even those with the same genes, are much more responsive to instruction and exposure. These differences may reflect natural variations in the way the brain functions. In practice, some children respond much better than others to instruction, for reasons we do not fully understand.

## WHAT'S GOING ON IN THE BRAIN?

The reading brain depends on several specialized networks or circuits in the front, middle, and back parts of its language hemisphere, which for most people is the left side of the cerebral cortex (the large, convoluted mass of gray matter that sits on the surface of the brain). Neuroscientists have been able to watch the reading brain at work without the patient experiencing any discomfort or loss of consciousness through scientific studies that use functional magnetic resonance imaging (fMRI), positron emission tomography (PET), magneto enchephalography (MEG), and electroencephalography (EEG).

Children with reading disabilities typically show a different pattern of brain activation from normally progressing young readers. Children with dyslexia have been found in some studies to process visual information more slowly. While dyslexia is a language-based learning disability, it is possible that the visual system abnormalities and reading disorders may coexist due to impairment of a common underlying neural system. Just because the recognition and interpretation of visual-print information is slow, for example, we cannot assume that a reading problem is primarily due to a visual processing abnormality. A common finding across laboratories is underactivation of the visual region in the back of the brain (occipital area) where visual images of words are recognized and stored, in both children and adults with dyslexia. Still other studies report that the front of the brain (frontal lobe), associated with speech production and speech sound awareness, is overactive in the dyslexic person who is still laboriously sounding out words. Many studies are in agreement that dyslexia is associated with reduced activation in the areas at the junction of three of the four major lobes (the parietal, occipital, and temporal lobes of the left hemisphere). Significantly, the poor reader seems to have trouble integrating the activity of brain regions responsible for different parts of the reading task.

The results of some fMRI studies have also shown that children whose left cerebral hemispheres are not functioning normally for reading may try to compensate for the problem by activating regions of the right cerebral hemisphere. In proficient readers, those regions remain relatively (as compared to controls) inactive during the reading task. Such patterns have been observed in adults and children with reading disabilities.

Continued study will likely provide even more brain-based explanations for reading difficulties. However, one of the most important findings of cognitive neuroscience is that the abnormal brain activation patterns of a young dyslexic reader can be somewhat "normalized" through excellent remedial instruction. If instruction is sufficiently intense and directed at the underlying language process-ing problems involving speech sounds, letter sequences, automatic recognition of whole words, and fluent reading for meaning, then the back regions of the brain take on more responsibility for processing print. This is as it should be, because the person who reads with fluency primarily activates the back part of the brain. Back (occipital) re-gions of the brain are most closely associated with accu-rate, automatic recognition of words in print.

In conclusion, cognitive neuroscience and genetics have enabled us to understand that children with reading disabilities have disruptions in the neurological mecha-nisms that underlie reading. The location and some of the dynamics of those disruptions have been discovered, along with their consequences for reading behavior. The neuro-logical disruptions are, in most cases, a consequence of ge-netic influences whose operation is not thoroughly understood at this time. However, the findings of neuro-science are converging very well with research findings from psychology and education, and have led us to un-derstand why effective reading instruction must contain several essential components and characteristics.

# 6

# EXPERT TEACHING

## Is the Treatment

## DO REGULAR CLASS PROGRAMS
## MAKE A DIFFERENCE?

So many children struggle with reading—in some schools, more than half are in the "at risk" category on tests that predict later reading achievement—that it is not reasonable to expect reading specialists and special educators to provide all the necessary instruction. If children do not receive appropriate instruction until they are referred to a specialist, many precious months of instructional time are lost. Early intervention, in kindergarten and first grade, is less expensive, more effective, and easier to deliver than remediation delivered later. The referral rate of children to special and remedial services is greatly reduced in public school systems if children receive preventative instruction from the regular classroom teacher that is consistent with the findings of scientific reading research. Regular classroom programs can make a big difference in reducing the number of children who eventually need special services.

## FIVE ESSENTIAL COMPONENTS OF EFFECTIVE READING PROGRAMS

The essential characteristics and components of effective classroom reading instruction are no longer a matter of serious debate. Research-based reading instruction is now defined in the appropriation bills of several federally funded programs, including the Reading First program of No Child Left Behind. Reading First has provided funding to low performing schools to improve reading achievement. Since Reading First's implementation in 2002, many eligible schools have raised reading achievement in high-risk populations using research-based instructional programs. Policy makers could require the implementation of good reading instruction practices because a strong research consensus had already identified what works best for children at risk. That consensus emerged from the *National Reading Panel Report* in 2000 and in many subsequent books and papers by leading scientists. Reading instruction that aligned with research findings includes, at a minimum, five essential components or ingredients found to support reading success:

- *Phonemic awareness*—the ability to recognize, remember, and manipulate the individual sounds (phonemes) in spoken words. Phonemic awareness is the understanding that phonemes are blended in spoken words and can be broken apart (segmented). For example, the word *tap* can be separated into three component sounds or phonemes: /t/, /a/, and /p/. Phonemic awareness is a necessary underlying skill for mapping alphabetic symbols to spoken words. It can be developed through instruction. Some children develop this awareness readily, and others need intensive, direct instruction to do so. If a child has not yet developed phonemic awareness, trying to teach him or her phonics and the concept of the alphabetic principle can be frustrating and lead to failure.

• *Phonics and word recognition*—knowledge of the predictable correspondences between phonemes and graphemes (the letters and letter combinations that represent phonemes). Although English is less predictable than some other languages, with mastery of the sound-symbol relationships and knowledge of word meaning and origin, English is highly predictable. Only about 4% of English words are truly irregular. Readers use phonics as they learn to recognize words accurately and automatically, to decode unfamiliar words, and to spell. A good command of phonics helps a child to memorize less predictable words that must be memorized and to automatically recognize decodable words such as *sit*. When children begin to blend and break apart words using actual letters, they are starting to master phonics. Explicit and systematic instruction in phonics helps all children read and spell more accurately and fluently than non-phonics instruction. Researchers have found that phonics instruction is very important for preventing reading failure in children at risk.

- *Reading fluency*—reading text with sufficient speed and accuracy to support comprehension. Fluency can be enhanced with various instructional techniques, such as repeated timed readings of grade appropriate text and with reading practice. To comprehend well, students must achieve adequate oral reading fluency rates. Fluency is represented by words correct per minute (WCPM) on a 1-minute or 2-minute timed reading of a passage. Thresholds for adequate oral reading fluency from 1st to 8th grade are well established by research, as shown in Table 1.

- *Vocabulary development*—knowledge of the individual word meanings in a text and those meanings learned by repeated exposure to a word's use in context and by explicit, direct instruction of definitions. Reading comprehension depends heavily on vocabulary development. Providing more familiar synonyms and antonyms is helpful. Modeling the use of the word in different, easily understood sentences is also an effec-

**Table 1.** Oral Reading Fluency Thresholds for Grades 1 to 8

| GRADE | PERCENTILE | FALL WCPM | WINTER WCPM | SPRING WCPM |
|---|---|---|---|---|
| 1 | 50 | -- | 23 | 53 |
| 2 | 50 | 51 | 72 | 89 |
| 3 | 50 | 71 | 92 | 107 |
| 4 | 50 | 94 | 112 | 123 |
| 5 | 50 | 110 | 127 | 139 |
| 6 | 50 | 127 | 140 | 150 |
| 7 | 50 | 128 | 136 | 150 |
| 8 | 50 | 133 | 146 | 151 |

*Note: Data are derived from Hasbrouck and Tindal (2006).*

tive strategy. Creating graphic representations, such as diagrams and conceptual maps, with children can help to teach vocabulary, as well as relationships between words, categories, and concepts. Reading and increasing background knowledge in a wide range of topics are the best ways to increase vocabulary. It is important that readers understand the meaning of most of the words or comprehension is compromised. Therefore, children must learn many new words at home and at school. Book readings and discussions, science and social studies activities, field trips, and informal discussions, are all great activities for learning new words. Parents can help by reading books to their children that are specifically written to build vocabulary, such as children's word books and any other books that introduce new vocabulary. When reading to their children, parents have an excellent opportunity to explain multiple meanings of words and common idioms and metaphors often used in children's books. Parents should use interesting vocabulary whenever possible when conversing with their children and encourage them to ask about the meanings of words they do not know.

- *Reading comprehension*—Comprehension skills and strategies, background knowledge, and verbal reasoning are all employed by good readers to understand, remember, and communicate what has been read. Good readers read with purpose and flexibility. Teachers can be instrumental in teaching children the skills and strategies necessary to navigate narrative and expository texts. Early on, readers should be taught to interact actively with the text. In preschool, this means having children demonstrate understanding by engaging in a variety of play activities, by retelling and reenacting stories, and by answering literal questions. Children should be making connections to prior knowledge and be encouraged to predict what might happen next in the story. While comprehension skill development in preschool is done mainly through oral discussion and play activities, in kindergarten, children are beginning to record their understandings of character and to create problem and solution charts. By first grade, students can demonstrate their understanding through graphic organizers (i.e., visual images or charts that compare concepts). Research has shown that children who are taught to recognize story structure, including the content and organization of stories, understand and remember the stories better. A child should begin learning how to summarize informational texts and to retell stories in the primary grades. The child's skills in this area should continue to develop as he or she progresses through the grades. Likewise, parents and teachers should use progressively more challenging questions and questions that are open ended and inferential in nature as children progress through the grades. For children with comprehension difficulties, there is no substitute for daily practice with the skills described above, directed by a teacher or by a computer program that provides interpretive assistance and immediate feedback to the student.

In addition to the essential five components named in federal laws, many reading experts agree that two more should be added:

- *Basic writing skills*—the ability to compose and tran-
  scribe conventional English with accuracy, fluency,
  and clarity of expression. Writing is dependent on
  many language skills and processes and is often even
  more problematic for children than reading. Writing is
  a language discipline with many component skills that
  must be directly taught. Because writing demands
  using different skills at the same time, such as generating language, spelling, handwriting, and using capital-
  ization and punctuation, it puts a significant demand
  on working memory and attention. Thus, a student
  may demonstrate mastery of these individual skills,
  but when asked to integrate all of them at once, mastery of an individual skill, such as handwriting, often
  deteriorates. To write on demand, a student has to
  have mastered, to the point of being automatic, each
  skill involved.

- *Comprehending and using spoken language*—the ability to
  listen and understand the meaning of what someone
  is saying, use grammatical English in academic set-
  tings, and formulate and express ideas orally. Oral
  language is the foundation for literacy and facilitates
  the ability to comprehend and communicate the goals
  of reading and writing.

## EFFECTIVE TEACHING

The essential components of instruction should be delivered
by a well-trained teacher who knows how to use a well-
designed, validated approach or program. A partnership between Newgrange Education Center (based in Princeton,
New Jersey) and the Trenton, New Jersey public schools

provides a good example of how well-informed teachers can make a difference. Newgrange currently assists in kindergarten and first grade classes at five schools that have some of the lowest reading scores in the district.

Newgrange Education Center and the Trenton public schools developed a productive relationship that allowed all parties to learn new teaching practices. The teachers in Trenton learned to implement the five essential components of an effective reading program. They also used test data to identify students who were in need of remediation. Teachers, administrators, and other staff members in the Trenton Public School District worked as partners with the staff of Newgrange to transform their practice. The reading ability of students has increased significantly since the partnership began.

## PROGRAMS

In addition to supporting and training skilled teachers, such as those at Newgrange Education Center, good programs are essential to helping children with their reading difficulties. Publishers of regular classroom reading programs have made tremendous improvements in the design of their materials over the last 10 years, but only some of them have been studied under controlled research conditions. Sources now exist to help schools select the strongest programs, including the website of the Florida Center for Reading Research (*www.fcrr.org*) and the What Works Clearinghouse of the Institute for Education Sciences in the United States Department of Education (*www.whatworks.ed.gov*). The International Dyslexia Association's website (*www.interdys.org*) also provides links to information about preventive and remedial programs, as well as the teacher training programs that support successful implementation. Many of these resources are listed in Chapter 10 of this book.

If the regular classroom instructional program is skillfully delivered, and extra small group instruction (4–6 students) is given to children who are only somewhat behind their peers, the number of children who remain below average in basic reading skill can be reduced to 6–10%. Those children usually need more intensive, specialized instruction, such as described in Chapter 7. But regardless of whether the program is for the regular classroom or something more specialized, the consistent finding from large-scale research in schools is that all components of instruction must be taught well, and those components should be integrated with one another.

For example, if children need to learn to identify speech sounds in words, then speech sound awareness should be a part of phonics and spelling instruction. When phonics is taught, children must apply what they have learned during reading and writing of meaningful material. When reading fluency is the goal, comprehension must be emphasized and never sacrificed for the sake of reading faster. When comprehension is the goal, written responses solidify learning. Integrated lessons flow logically from one component to the next and do not emphasize some to the exclusion of others.

## INSTRUCTION

Not only the content of the program, but also the style of teaching, make a significant difference in the success of the student at risk for reading difficulty. Instruction that is most likely to help poor readers in the classroom is

- *Explicit*—Each language and print concept is clearly and directly explained by the teacher, rather than left to discovery through incidental encounters with information. Poor readers do not learn that print represents speech simply from exposure to books or print.

- *Systematic*—The entire system of speech sounds, spelling patterns, sentence structures, text genres, and language conventions is taught rather than a few bits of information here and there as topics happen to arise.

- *Cumulative*—Children are given continual review, as one skill builds on another.

- *Multisensory*—Children are actively engaged in learning language concepts and other information, often by using their hands, arms, mouths, eyes, and whole bodies while learning. For example, students read aloud and act out dialogue among characters in a story or say spelling words slowly while they write them on a rough surface, such as a carpet or sand tray. A multisensory math activity would be learning fractions by measuring and constructing a model of a building.

- *Sequential and Incremental*—Instruction proceeds in manageable steps. The teacher follows a scope and sequence of skills to ensure coverage of all essential concepts for reading and writing.

- *Data-driven*—What the teacher emphasizes, where the teacher gives extra help, and how fast the teacher proceeds with the small groups are determined by the results of progress-monitoring assessments. Curriculum-based measurements, such as oral reading fluency tests and brief measures of skill retention and application, are essential for guiding the content and emphasis of instruction.

However, even when appropriate reading instruction is delivered with an effective style of teaching, children may have difficulties. Thus, additional strategies for managing language and listening problems in the classroom may be needed.

## MANAGEMENT OF LANGUAGE AND LISTENING PROBLEMS IN THE CLASSROOM

Dyslexic students with attentional problems can easily lose focus in the presence of background noise and other distractions. They may be overwhelmed by too many visual, auditory, or social stimuli. They often have trouble remaining focused on and remembering directions and information given by the teacher. The following adaptations in classroom management and teacher behavior can be very helpful:

- Support verbal directions and information with visual information (e.g., writing, pictures, charts, modeling directions)
- Maintain eye contact and keep the child close
- Rephrase if the child does not understand or remember
- Teach key vocabulary before studying a topic
- Alternate movement with periods of seat-work

- Check student understanding by asking for verbal responses
- Make tasks meaningful by connecting them to life experience
- Teach memory strategies, such as categorizing and mental rehearsal, and encourage their use
- Restate and emphasize major ideas

The International Dyslexia Association is concerned that many teachers are licensed without knowing the content and procedures of preventive classroom reading instruction outlined above. Teachers usually need considerable professional development, classroom coaching, and administrative support to deliver instruction effectively. This investment pays off, however, because preventive reading instruction greatly reduces the costs of special education services and greatly improves the school experience of a large number of children at risk.

# 7

# SEVERE DYSLEXIA

## and Other Learning Disabilities

## WHAT ARE SEVERE READING DISABILITIES?

Children with the most severe dyslexia are those who score below the 10th percentile on reading tests, in spite of normal classroom instruction. For research purposes, studies of poor readers include students who score anywhere from the 5th to the 30th percentile on reading tests. These children may or may not have IQ scores that are significantly higher than their reading scores. Federal and state laws in the past required that to qualify for special education services students had to have a "severe discrepancy" between their IQ and their reading achievement, but researchers have shown that the nature and characteristics of a serious reading problem are not predicted by a student's IQ. IQ testing may provide information about a student's intellectual strengths and weaknesses that is helpful for counseling and teaching purposes, but it does not predict how readily a student will respond to reading instruction, or tell us anything significant about the nature of a student's reading disorder.

Emily and John are two students whose difficulties with reading illustrate this point. Emily's overall cognitive ability was in the very superior or gifted range. Her general language skills were determined to be in the very superior range, as well. However, her basic pre-reading skills, although generally high average, were below expectation based on her exceptionally strong language and cognitive abilities. Students such as Emily, with high IQs, are very noticeable because their reading problem stands out among their other strengths, and because they tend to have high academic aspirations in spite of their inability to read and write proficiently. Emily would not qualify for special education services in most public schools, although her problem would inhibit her achievement of high academic aspirations.

John, on the other hand, seemed to have difficulty in all aspects of speech and language. Students with low average IQs and students who, like John, show no significant discrepancies between IQ and achievement, are just as deserving of—and in need of—remedial academic instruction. Unfortunately, these students with low average ability and poor reading skills often get overlooked for reading intervention and may be the victims of low academic expectations. John would not qualify for special education services, but he would be eligible for supportive and remedial intervention in a school that follows a "tiered" approach to instruction under a response-to-intervention (RTI) model of service.

Children with the most severe reading disabilities often, but not always, have a family history of dyslexia. The neurobiological nature of their difficulty becomes obvious when, in spite of excellent instruction, they make slow progress and have trouble retaining what they have learned about reading and spelling the printed word. It is estimated that 30% of those with dyslexia have coexisting attention-deficit/hyperactivity disorder (AD/HD). If a child has both dyslexia and AD/HD, both the reading disability and the attentional/behavioral problems must be treated if the child is to flourish and meet his or her academic potential. Children with more than one kind of problem tend to be those who qualify for special education services. Boys are referred for special services about four times more often than girls because they have a higher incidence of attention and behavior problems, even though the ratio of boys to girls who have reading problems is only about three to two.

## ATTEMPTS TO HELP EMILY AND JOHN

Sometimes early identification of a reading problem and a well-supported approach to intervention is not enough. Even though Emily received direct instruction in a well-designed, research-based, early reading intervention program that developed phonemic awareness skills, mastery of the alphabetic principle, and reading fluency, she was not progressing. Because Emily and her progress were frequently evaluated and carefully observed, her teachers and parents identified problems with maintaining attention, distractibility, and impulsive behavior, so she was diagnosed with AD/HD.

John also did not respond to early intervention services. Although he was exposed to phonics, for example, the phonic elements were not introduced systematically. Without adequate practice, he was never able to achieve mastery. His unreliable memory compounded by memory retrieval problems made reading and writing a guessing game rather than a demonstration of mastery of the alphabetic principle. It wasn't until John's parents moved him to a school that specialized in teaching children with dyslexia that he began to make progress.

For children such as Emily and John, the first attempt to address reading difficulties may not be enough. In other cases, the intervention may be the best instruction for a particular child but progress is very slow. It can be challenging for parents and educators to know what to expect.

## WHAT IS THE LONG-TERM PROGRESS
## OF STUDENTS WITH READING DISABILITIES?

The National Institutes of Health and the United States Department of Education, along with other institutions and foundations, have sponsored a series of long-term studies of students' reading growth and the factors that account for successful outcomes. Various approaches to remediation and aspects of instruction have been compared. Students with severe reading disabilities and students with milder forms of reading problems have been the subjects of long-term research on the causes and treatments of reading failure.

Research that examines the relative effects of different programs and methods is called *intervention* or *treat-*

*ment research.* Newer studies are addressing RTI as a factor in understanding how severe a student's dyslexia might be. The first important finding of a series of scientifically conducted studies on RTI is that most students with reading disabilities can be taught to read, at least adequately, and many can become proficient readers. Younger students who are identified as at risk when screened can make significant progress with 30–40 minutes of remedial or preventive instruction per day. Only the most severe reading problems require one-on-one tutoring; most students with milder problems can progress just as well if there are 3–5 students in a group. Older students (beyond third grade) require much more instructional time (up to 2 hours per day) to overcome a reading problem.

Effective intervention programs have all the instructional principles and components listed in Chapter 6 and later in this chapter, but the relative emphasis on those components varies somewhat from program to program. For example, some programs emphasize teaching the speech sounds of English in great depth, while others require more time on text reading and language comprehension. In spite of differences among programs and approaches, students' rate of progress in basic reading skills is remarkably similar across studies that have monitored reading growth of students at risk.

In general, students in good remedial programs with a strong phonics component will make the most progress in phonic decoding, compared to related skills, such as spelling or silent passage reading comprehension. Reading fluency, which is dependent on fast sight word recognition, is the most difficult skill to bring up to the average range, especially if a student's problem was identified after first or second grade. In other words, students who are very poor readers can make significant gains in basic reading skill relative to their peer group, but tend to remain slow readers. That is why some common and fair accommodations for students with reading disabilities are extra time on tests, shortened reading assignments, and supplementary use of audiotaped material so that time spent reading is kept within reason.

## WHAT TO EXPECT
## FROM AN INTERVENTION PROGRAM

A successful intervention for one child at any given moment might be very different from the intervention that works for another child or for the same child at another time. For an intervention to be effective, educators and others must frequently monitor a child's progress and make adjustments as needed for progress to continue. Emily and John had very different problems, so it is not surprising that the ideal interventions and the rate and extent of the progress they made were also different.

Once Emily's AD/HD was treated medically and educationally with accommodations, such as preferential seating, she started to progress academically. By the end of first grade, she was achieving in the low average to average range in all reading and writing areas. The goal for Emily will be for her to eventually read and write well above average because of her exceptional language skills. This should be a realistic goal because Emily exhibited only mild weaknesses in phonological awareness and her rapid naming skills were average. Phonological awareness and rapid naming are underlying language skills that are critical to beginning reading. Emily's solid academic progress should continue, as long as appropriate direct reading and writing instruction is provided, and her AD/HD is effectively treated.

Not surprisingly, dyslexic students who begin a remedial program with somewhat higher reading skills make more rapid progress in passage comprehension than the students who begin remediation with the lowest reading scores. Students who start with somewhat better reading skills are able to narrow the gap between themselves and their peers to a greater extent than students who start at the lowest levels of reading skill. Very few of the severely reading disabled students who are identified after third grade close the achievement gap altogether.

John, for example, would not be expected to make the same progress as Emily. John's progress certainly improved at his new school; however, his progress could still be considered slow and laborious. His progress was hindered by significant difficulties with rapid sight word recognition and dysfluent reading. These challenges compromised his reading comprehension. By the end of fifth grade, John was reading at an end of second-grade level. He depended heavily on assistive technology to remain abreast of reading and writing in his core subject areas. Yet, John was progressing in reading and writing and mastering grade-level content in his core classes. His parents were pleased because they felt that John had blossomed in many ways in the nurturing environment of his specialized school.

In most intervention studies, the most rapid gains are made within the first 12 hours of instruction; after that, progress continues, but the pace can seem very slow to students, parents, and teachers. Some students with the most severe reading disabilities need 2 to 3 years of intensive instruction to become functional readers. It is important for teachers and parents to expect slow, steady progress after the initial period of more rapid gains, and to avoid giving up prematurely.

No study of children with severe reading disabilities has claimed a cure for dyslexia. A small percentage of students (about 2–5%) appear to have chronic and severe problems learning to read for which we do not yet have effective treatments. These students are sometimes called *treatment resistors* because they do not improve even when expert instruction is delivered for weeks, months, and even years. Researchers are investigating the characteristics of the students who make very slow or limited progress in spite of excellent teaching. At the first-grade level, students with the most severe reading disabilities also have the most severe problems with phonemic awareness, rapid naming of objects, and writing the alphabet. Very poor spelling is one of the most accurate indicators of a severe reading disability at the first-grade level. In addition, pronounced weaknesses in phonic decoding of nonsense words, accurate reading of real words in lists, and overall reading scores are the most reliable indicators that a child may not respond readily to good instruction. The children who respond better to educational interventions in first and second grade tend to have higher verbal abilities in general, are more independent in their work habits, and are better able to focus on a given task until it is completed than the students who respond more poorly. Children who respond better to instruction also tend to have fewer behavior problems, better memory for verbal information, and higher vocabulary scores.

In the regular classroom, a well-implemented instructional program that is systematic and explicit, that targets phonological skills and alphabet knowledge, and that is teacher-directed can substantially reduce the number of students at risk for reading problems. If the regular class instruction is supplemented with small group instruction that bolsters specific skills in which children have been found to be weak, most children will succeed. About 75% of children with reading problems in first and second grade will respond well to intervention, and most of the time they will sustain their gains and progress at an average rate.

Children in the 2–5% of *treatment resistors* who respond more poorly to instruction and who remain substantially below grade level in reading may make better progress if several adjustments are made. These changes include spending more time in a strong remedial program, participating in more frequent lessons with continual reinforcement of learned skills, or making adjustments in methods. Children with the most severe problems often have coexisting problems with attention, behavior, emotional functioning, and/or organization in time and space. Many of these children will be eligible for special education and will need an IEP with reading, language, and writing goals, as well as goals in all other relevant areas.

According to recent scientific research, students who begin at the 5th percentile typically progress to about the 14th percentile if instruction is expert and intensive. Students who begin below the 16th percentile typically progress to the 35th percentile when the program is effective. These gains are commendable and are attained after many weeks of determined effort by both student and teacher. Although the gains do not usually result in children being able to read proficiently, or even at grade level, they do increase the student's chances of coping with academic assignments. If students with severe reading disabilities can attain a tenth-grade reading comprehension level, they can decipher most everyday reading material. Thus, reading at the tenth-grade reading level will open employment doors for many adults and enable them to independently read menus, fill out forms, read newspapers, navigate on a computer, and read instructions.

The results from research do not support the view that all children with severe dyslexia or reading disabilities should be able to read at grade level. They do support the importance of long-term, intensive, specialized instruction given with sufficient expertise and over a long enough period that children will demonstrate significant improvement.

## WHAT ARE THE CHARACTERISTICS OF EFFECTIVE INSTRUCTION FOR SEVERE READING DISABILITIES?

In addition to instruction that addresses the critical reading skills covered in Chapter 6, appropriate instruction for students with severe dyslexia includes the following:

- *Direct teaching to areas of need*—Students may vary somewhat in the extent to which they need instruction in the critical reading skills of phonological skills, language comprehension and expression, phonic decoding, text reading fluency, vocabulary, writing skills, and comprehension strategies, described in detail in Chapter 6. Comprehension skills and strategies must be taught directly, including summarizing, clarifying, predicting, and generating questions, with both narrative and informational text. When students cannot yet read, having someone read aloud to them, using technology-based reading tools, or playing audiotaped material can help them learn vocabulary and gain background knowledge.

- *Ample cumulative review*—Students often need what seems like an inordinate amount of review and practice to develop word recognition habits and other skills. Computer technology can help provide that practice, and curriculum-based measurement can help the teacher decide when enough practice has occurred.

- *Explicit presentation of language concepts*—Students benefit from understanding why words are spelled the way they are and from developing metalinguistic awareness—the ability to think about and reflect on language. Word games and word play can contribute to this awareness of language.

- *Transfer and application of what is learned*—Children with learning disabilities often need help applying what they have learned to new examples and new situations.

- *Flexible strategy use*—Effective instruction emphasizes strategies for deciphering written language and for problem solving in general. It includes talking aloud about thought processes and evaluating whether strategies have been used appropriately.

- *Linking of speaking, listening, reading, and writing*—The simultaneous use of these language functions reinforces concepts and promotes learning through all the senses. Children should spell and write words they have been taught to read. Written expression should be expected and supported even if students are poor at spelling and handwriting. Tasks can be highly structured to facilitate success.

## CLASSROOM ACCOMMODATIONS

Accommodations do not replace academic language therapy or remedial instruction. However, as students with severe reading disabilities move through school, many accommodations may be needed that will remove barriers caused by poor reading, writing, or study skills. Common accommodations for students with severe reading disabilities are the provision of taped texts, someone to read aloud, assistance with note-taking, extra time on tests, adaptation of course requirements, provision of technological aids, and assistance with hand-written work.

## CONTROVERSIAL THERAPIES

Independent, scientific studies of children with reading disabilities have not verified the claims of controversial therapies for reading involving colored lenses, vitamin doses, spinning and balance treatments, memory pills, creeping and crawling, sensory integration therapy, water ingestion, and the like. The treatment for a reading disability is direct, systematic, explicit, cumulative, incremental, and multisensory structured language teaching of the critical components of reading instruction. Most children with reading difficulties can progress to grade level, and the remaining 2–5% can and do make progress, but may never achieve mastery of grade level skills. However, appropriate remedial instruction should be provided to all of these children so that they may achieve the best possible academic outcome. Achieving the highest possible level of reading ability is an important educational goal for all children.

Often the work of educating dyslexic individuals is challenging for both students and teachers, but the rewards are plentiful. Students with dyslexia tend to succeed in the long run, especially when caring family members, friends, and teachers invest the time, effort, and skill in nurturing their abilities.

# 8

# EMOTIONAL CONSEQUENCES

## of Dyslexia and Other Reading Problems

## HOW DYSLEXIA AFFECTS EMOTIONAL DEVELOPMENT

The experience of being dyslexic can elicit a range of uncomfortable emotions in young and old alike. Even kindergarten children can be aware that they are not learning things that seem easy for others. Young children expect when they attend school that they will learn to read, write, and do math, and when they have difficulty, they are mystified. It is natural for them to attribute even minor academic problems to being "dumb" because they have no other way of understanding what might be wrong and no effective strategies for relieving their sense of inadequacy. In addition, the child may be very puzzled by the inconsistency of his or her memory and learning.

Parents and teachers may conclude that the child is not trying hard enough or is not motivated.

Many of these children experience a destructive emotional cycle that begins with an awareness of disappointing adults. Simultaneously, the child is also frustrated with him or herself. The feeling of inadequacy that results is very painful, especially because the child does not understand the difficulty that he or she is experiencing, and feels totally helpless to correct or avoid making mistakes that lead to academic failure. The shame of disappointing adults and disappointing oneself then turns to resentment of those who seem to hold unachievable expectations. This psychological trap—for which there seems no reasonable way out—leads alternately to anger at others and anger at oneself. Anger at oneself, in turn, can quickly be transformed into a chronic sense of helplessness and even depression.

Dyslexic individuals often experience high levels of anxiety. Anxiety is fear of the unknown and worry that one will not be able to meet the expectations of others. It is closely related to having no sense of control over what will happen next and chronic feelings of helplessness. Anxiety is a predictable response to dyslexia, because the person is never sure how the difficulty will affect performance and whether embarrassment or failure lies ahead. Some children become fearful of school and seek to avoid it because the anxiety triggered there is extremely uncomfortable. When the child is extremely anxious, it is more difficult if not impossible for him or her to pay attention, concentrate, and stay on task. Some children come to believe (usually unconsciously) that they have little control over their own learning process.

Early detection of dyslexia and early intervention usually alleviate and prevent emotional problems such as anxiety that make reading and schoolwork even more difficult. Children are less anxious if they understand what is happening to them, are receiving support, and are building confidence by accomplishing tasks and making progress.

Problems can emerge in families of dyslexic children as family members struggle to provide the extra support the child needs. Parents may have to spend hours each evening helping their dyslexic child with homework. Many parents read material aloud that the child cannot read independently. It may also be necessary for parents to write or type assignments for their child. The demand this assistance places on the parent-child relationship can be enormous, and it reduces the opportunity for the parent and child to enjoy each other in other, less stressful ways. The extra time spent with the dyslexic child also takes parental time away from other children in the family who may become resentful. And, the extra time and support that is intended to help the child with dyslexia may actually result in the child feeling inadequate and helpless.

Social problems can also arise. About 30% of dyslexic children also have at least a mild form of AD/HD, and consequently are less organized, self-controlled, and conforming to social rules than their peers. Such behaviors may be alienating to others. In addition, dyslexic students' difficulty with language may be a turn-off to peers and may foster miscommunication. And, students who feel badly about themselves may not have the social confidence or skill to seek and maintain friendships and may become withdrawn or alienated from their friends and families.

# MINIMIZING THE IMPACT OF DYSLEXIA

The impact of dyslexia on individuals depends on the severity of the problem, the presence or absence of other problems, the person's temperament and emotional resilience, and the nature and timeliness of the instruction the person receives. It also depends on the person's emotional support system. Studies of resilience in children with learning disabilities have shown that three major factors determine whether a person ultimately makes a good emotional and social adjustment in school and life:

- The person's ability to solve problems and navigate in spite of the learning difficulty

- A strength that provides success and self-esteem

- A strong, constant, supportive relationship with at least one adult who believes in the child's worth and capabilities

## *Ability to Solve Problems*

Problem-solving ability refers to the person's resourcefulness and flexibility in dealing with obstacles, whether they are academic, emotional, or social. For example, the person who writes poorly can cope with that frustration more readily if he or she is willing to accept feedback, ask for proofreading help, start assignments early, learn to dictate, and acknowledge the problem openly with teachers or supervisors. The student who is hurt by the critical comments of uninformed teachers can channel that experience into effective self-advocacy, learning to inform others about his or her problems and needs. The student who does not comprehend information can pursue clarification instead of withdrawing from a task.

Helen, for example, experienced social communication problems that she eventually learned to handle. Like many dyslexic individuals, Helen had significant expressive language difficulties. Her quiet and reserved demeanor did not reveal the extent of her social anxiety and feelings of difference. On the surface, Helen was painfully shy, and Helen's mother reported that she really did not have friends outside of school. The origin of her social shyness, however, was a lack of basic communication skills expected in her high school peer group. She was slow to respond to questions, seldom initiated conversation, and had trouble formulating sentences that were syntactically correct and clear. She was afraid to ask her teachers to clarify a homework assignment and did not feel confident to call a classmate for help.

Helen's tutor was in communication with school personnel to maximize her organizational support. Helen worked with her tutor to set up an assignment calendar that helped her to plan for long-term assignments and to organize, generate, and edit essays and other writing assignments. The goal of Helen's support was to have her become more and more independent. Gradually, Helen began initiating social communication on her own, and she became an increasingly stronger student, learning how to study and to organize her academic responsibilities much more independently.

## Development of Strengths

Dyslexic people with compensatory strengths, interests, and talents have a better chance to salvage their self-esteem and enjoy social relationships. Areas of strength or interest may include mathematical or technology pursuits, artistic talents, musical skills, community service, athletic teams, or mechanical and spatial projects. Often these interests and pursuits are somewhat unconventional and may be trying or costly for parents to support, but they are therapeutic for children.

Some dyslexic people are highly gifted and talented in areas other than reading and writing. Others are of average ability, and still others struggle with almost everything in school and outside of school. Nevertheless, a parent's willingness to develop an interest with the child and to pursue it together can be very helpful. Non-academic pursuits, including simple recreational activities, outdoor adventures, or volunteer work can be an important vehicle for learning goal-setting, self-discipline, and realistic self-assessment. Thus, it is important for parents and teachers to identify an area in which, with hard work and coaching, a child can learn to at least enjoy a reasonable level of competence and success, and perhaps, learn to excel. The dyslexic students in the following case studies relied on strengths and talents other than reading and writing that helped them develop self-esteem.

- Molly was a dyslexic student with special athletic talent. Although she could dance elegantly and with ease, she could barely write legibly or control pencil movements while she formed letters. Her natural physical gifts, which emerged in sports, dance, and gymnastics, bolstered her sense of self-worth even while she struggled with reading and language.

- Tom, a tenth grade student reading on a fifth-grade level before starting an intensive educational program, was a natural athlete. In addition, Tom was a natural leader among his peers. Socially adept from early childhood, he became captain of his ice-hockey team.

- Jennie spent years remediating her dyslexia, and she was extremely sensitive about her academic challenges. She resisted her mother's attempts to support her, preferring not to recognize the impact her dyslexia was having on her performance in academic classes. Jennie habitually challenged her tutors, often appearing very negative and resisting instruction. Art was her true passion. Her high school art teacher commented that Jennie was one of the most gifted artists he had ever taught. Over time, as Jennie was encouraged to explore her interest and talent in painting, she also became a strong reader. Her entire demeanor changed as she progressed through school, from sad and self-conscious in middle school, to confident and self-assured in high school. Jennie's strong visual-perceptual skills allowed her to pursue a college degree with an art major.

## Supportive Adults

A supportive relationship with a family member or someone outside the family can make a great difference to the dyslexic student's self-understanding and self-esteem. A supportive and nurturing adult is a good listener who can help the dyslexic student recognize and verbalize his or her feelings. He or she will help the child identify areas of strength, set realistic goals, solve problems constructively, and recognize small improvements when they occur. This person might be a parent, an athletic coach, a caring teacher, a leader in a church youth group, or a psychological counselor.

Homework is an important opportunity for a parent or sibling to provide support. However, it can also upend family routines and family harmony. Homework assignments often trigger fear, anxiety, and feelings of being overwhelmed in the dyslexic student. Teachers expect that students can manage homework on their own, but in reality, parents and siblings of dyslexic students often need to provide structure, strategies, encouragement, information, and other forms of assistance. How can the stress of this situation be minimized?

- *Communicate with each other*. Determine the specifics of the assignment, the expectations for its presentation, and when it is due. Stay in touch with the teacher, not only to find out what is required, but also to report any specific issues related to the child's ability to complete assigned tasks. Before the child sits down to work, go over the task together and strategize how to accomplish it.

- *Get organized*. Keep an assignment notebook. Buy pocket inserts for completed assignments and other material. Keep a daily, weekly, and monthly schedule in the notebook. Schedule time with the child for homework and breaks. Schedule other activities, too. Put hard tasks before easier or more pleasurable ones. Keep a special place clear, well lit, reasonably quiet, and comfortable for work that requires concentration. Have a well-supplied toolbox with office supplies.

Keep an extra set of textbooks at home, if possible, in case the first set is misplaced or left at school.

- *Strategize together.* Look over the specifics of an assignment with the child before he or she begins the work. Scan for easier and more difficult aspects of the task and plan an approach with the child. Determine an order for completing the assigned tasks. Help the child get started and then encourage the child to ask questions if he or she feels off track.

- *Model strategies.* Many teachers model good learning strategies such as the use of graphic organizers, underlining, and two-column note-taking. Find out which strategies the child's teachers are using in school and make sure that the child uses these good learning strategies at school and at home.

Providing so much extra time and support will be easier and more rewarding for some parents than others. In many families with a dyslexic child, the mother plays the role of the supportive nurturing adult. Many mothers have gone on to take intensive training in effective instructional techniques for teaching dyslexic children. This training has sometimes led to new careers for these mothers, where they find themselves teaching and supporting other dyslexic children besides their own.

In some families, however, dyslexia creates immense challenges for the family, and particularly the dyslexic child. Some parents who are themselves dyslexic feel guilt and shame, sensing that they are responsible for their child's academic difficulties. Rather than helping their child to set realistic goals and solve problems, some parents choose to delay recognition of their child's difficulties, hoping the early signs of dyslexia will disappear as the child ages. These parents may be intimidated by, afraid of, or resistant to the school's attempts to intervene early to help their child. Other parents who are not dyslexic but who may have seen a dyslexic sibling suffer without appropriate help, may react in an angry manner, recalling the pain of that sibling and the helplessness of the family. It is hard for these adults to realize that with early intervention, effective teaching, and appropriate accommodations, the academic outlook for dyslexic children today can be much more positive than it was when they were young. Far more information is available today that can minimize the impact of dyslexia on the child and his or her family.

## WHEN TO GET PROFESSIONAL HELP

Students with reading and other academic difficulties, whether or not they qualify for special education services, may need supportive or therapeutic psychological counseling or psychiatric treatment. The most common, treatable mental health problem associated with dyslexia is depression. While all children have periods of unhappiness, in most cases those feelings will pass. Depression is recognized in children by the following recurring and chronic symptoms:

- Negative and self-critical thoughts

- Depressed mood, lack of enjoyment

- Inability to imagine a positive future; feelings of helplessness and hopelessness

Psychotherapy, coupled with appropriate educational services, and perhaps medication, can relieve these symptoms. If a student expresses suicidal thoughts, becomes extremely withdrawn, is unable to concentrate or pay attention even when he or she wishes to, or has disturbed eating or sleeping patterns, additional psychiatric assessment should be obtained immediately. It is important that the therapist understands the emotional and psychological consequences of a learning disorder, and the role that educational treatment must play in the healing process. It may also be necessary for the therapist to monitor the student's academic progress to determine if appropriate accommodations are in place, that gains are being made, and to assist the family as an advocate for the child. If coexisting disorders such as AD/HD, anxiety, and depression are present, it is critical that these disorders be treated, or the remediation of the child's dyslexia will likely be limited and his or her emotional well-being compromised.

Shauna's story provides a fairly typical example of the ways in which a learning disorder can interact with emotional consequences. Shauna's dyslexia became evident early because she was essentially a nonreader when she started second grade. One teacher was especially instrumental in teaching Shauna how to read and nurturing her self-esteem.

In sixth grade, Shauna was diagnosed with a nonhyperactive attention disorder for which she received medical treatment. Nevertheless, academics became more and more challenging for her in middle school. With her organizational and attentional difficulties compounding her dyslexia, school was overwhelming. By seventh grade, Shauna was diagnosed with depression. She was treated with both medication and counseling to overcome her feelings of sadness and hopelessness.

In high school, Shauna finally developed effective coping strategies and began to realize her strengths. The first of these was self-understanding. Shauna once reflected, "To remain positive, you have to know who you are. You can't succeed with a negative attitude. You are not mentally or emotionally in a place where learning can happen. Being negative takes so much energy." The second coping strategy was the adoption of effective management of her demanding academic schedule. For example, Shauna used her superior verbal skills to aid her memory. She studied vocabulary words by saying them out loud and using them in sentences and used self-talk to teach herself new concepts. Shauna also adopted organizational routines, such as reviewing class notes daily. She learned to focus on her verbal gifts and planned a career as a lawyer to take advantage of those strengths.

Dyslexic students may experience complex challenges academically, socially, and emotionally, but with an appropriate academic program, help in developing areas of strength and interest, the emotional support of caring adults, and, sometimes, professional treatment by a psychologist, most will successfully cope with those challenges.

# 9

# A LIFE STORY

Jessica has dyslexia. Her story illustrates how one student met and coped with the many challenges of dyslexia from preschool to adulthood. Many of her experiences will be familiar to other people with dyslexia and their families. Jessica's strong intellectual gifts, willingness to work hard, and well-honed academic and study skills helped her not only to succeed, but also to excel.

When Jessica started preschool at age 3, school was already a challenge. Her preschool teacher raised concerns about Jessica's listening skills and her ability to concentrate. Jessica tended to wander off and begin playing by herself after playing only a few minutes with other children. She took a long time to complete her work and often needed help from the teacher.

From the beginning, Jessica struggled with learning to read. In particular, she had difficulty sounding out words and memorizing a vocabulary of basic sight words. She continued to be inattentive and had trouble completing assignments in kindergarten and first grade. Jessica's first-grade teacher told Jessica's mother that there was something wrong, but the teacher didn't know what was keeping Jessica from progressing as expected.

In second grade, Jessica was still having difficulty learning to read and write, and she scored poorly on standardized tests. Her mother was upset by a failing social studies test grade, knowing that Jessica had studied the material covered by the test the night before. Jessica's teacher wrote in big, red letters on the test, "58%—You did not pass." This unfortunate incident motivated Jessica's mother to have Jessica evaluated privately. Jessica underwent a psychoeducational evaluation, which is an assessment of her intellectual and cognitive abilities and academic achievement.

Jessica was found to be very bright and to have overall intellectual abilities in the superior range. Her academic achievement testing revealed significant weaknesses in reading decoding, reading comprehension, mathematical calculation, written expression, and spelling. At that time, Jessica's reading was described as labored, and she struggled to remember basic sight words. Her ability to sound out words was also poor. In addition, she scored below average in listening comprehension and oral expression skills on a speech and language evaluation. Jessica's mother shared the results of this evaluation with the school personnel. They found that Jessica was eligible for learning disability support services in math, reading, written expression, listening comprehension, and oral expression.

In addition to receiving direct instruction in these areas, Jessica's evaluation team recommended accommodations that included shortening, simplifying, and breaking down assignments into clearly defined steps. Jessica's teachers were advised to avoid multistep directions and to make sure that Jessica could repeat the directions in her own words. Preferential seating was another suggestion. Jessica often needed additional time to respond to oral questions and processed aural information more slowly. It was suggested that Jessica might need extra physical breaks between academic tasks to relieve tension and frustration. Multisensory techniques were also recommended to include tactile experiences in conjunction with aural and visual input.

Jessica's IEP (Individual Educational Program) was started in third grade. Her mother recalls that the IEP was presented in a positive and motivating manner to Jessica, and the staff met Jessica's specific needs, goals, and objectives. Her mother also commented that Jessica's headaches, upset stomachs, and resistance to school were replaced by pride in her school achievements.

Although Jessica was never formally diagnosed with an attention disorder, it was around third grade when she started taking medication to improve her ability to focus and sustain attention. She remained on medication until high school, when she stopped taking it because of the side effects.

In seventh grade, Jessica recalls being a reluctant reader. In fact, her basic reading skills were still a year below grade level, so that reading her textbooks was hard work. Jessica's mother bought another set of textbooks so Jessica could write in and highlight them. Jessica also recalls that even when she tried, she didn't achieve what she considered to be good grades. She described being frustrated by the challenge of reading, and how she really wanted to be a more independent and successful student. By this time, her mother was pursuing advanced study in a multisensory structured language program that she felt would be ideal for Jessica. She started tutoring Jessica in this program, which helped Jessica overcome the basic reading challenges that still plagued her.

In ninth grade, Jessica was reevaluated by her public school district. Areas of weakness for which she continued to qualify for the learning disabilities support program included word retrieval, verbal memory, listening comprehension, phonological processing, and math calculation. She received individual and small group instruction four times per week for 50 minutes each time. For the first time, Jessica's IEP included the provision of instruction in the multisensory, structured reading program that her mother had begun and that was completed by her special education teacher. Although Jessica found note-taking support helpful, she learned the importance of taking her own notes and used that strategy to study for tests.

Jessica learned effective learning strategies, took advantage of time-saving technology, and benefited from accommodations and modifications provided by her IEP. She found it helpful to take note cards and a calculator into tests because of her word retrieval and memory weaknesses. Preferential seating was also helpful. In fact, Jessica still prefers to sit in the front of the classroom. Jessica used a laptop for in-school essays and writing assignments, and she was not penalized for spelling errors on spontaneously written quizzes or writing assignments, unless she was using words from an assigned spelling list. However, spelling was included in the grade for final drafts of papers. She also benefited from the opportunity to hand in early drafts of papers to receive editing suggestions before she made the final revisions. All of these accommodations and modifications were listed on Jessica's IEP.

Jessica fondly remembers an excellent English teacher who spent over 2 years teaching her to write. This teacher taught her the structure of paragraphs and essays. With her teacher's guidance, Jessica also started using a writing rubric that included categories such as creativity, sentence structure, and mechanics on which she was rated on a four point scale. Jessica also learned the specific structure for writing a four or five paragraph essay. Her teacher taught her how to use transitional words, phrases and sentences, and proper wording to avoid awkward sentences. Jessica considered her significant improvement in writing as a major milestone.

During her high school career, Jessica became an increasingly competent and successful student. She started out getting Cs and Ds, but brought those grades up to As and Bs. Jessica studied American Sign Language (ASL) for 2 years instead of a foreign language and found that not only was she very successful, but she also really enjoyed the coursework. The academic area in which she feels she has struggled the most is math. Jessica took advantage of available math tutoring and actually began to tutor other students because she had a good grasp of the concepts.

Another major milestone for Jessica was becoming a recreational reader. By the end of high school, she started to read on her own, actually reading for pleasure. She was finally scoring in the average range on basic reading skills and above average on reading comprehension, although she was still a slow reader.

Jessica maintained a B average in a competitive high school. She received considerable recognition throughout her high school career for her hard work and dedication to academic improvement and excellence.

Jessica entered college with solid academic skills. Her freshman year, she took advantage of a peer tutoring program that helped her to edit her papers and further develop her writing. Math computation without the aid of pencil and paper was still a challenge, but she learned to write down everything and follow all the necessary steps to be successful. To study for her classes, Jessica used techniques that relied on her visual strengths, such as outlining, color coding, and adding shape cues to aid memory. She still needed extra time for reading, but she found that highlighting focused her attention and helped her remember what she had read.

Jessica was pleased that she had been able to use her American Sign Language with deaf children who were participating in a therapeutic riding program in which she was teaching, so she decided to study American Sign Language again in college. Unfortunately, the courses were not available. Studying a foreign language was not a requirement for her major, so she chose not to study one. Jessica learned how to manage her time and stay on top of her assignments, and how to advocate for herself. She became an excellent student.

Jessica's grades in college continued to improve, and by her senior year she had achieved a 4.0 grade point average for both semesters. She was also selected by her professors to receive an award honoring her outstanding achievement as an intervention specialist. Now in her twenties, Jessica has worked as a special educator for 2 years and is planning to apply to graduate school in occupational therapy. She wants to combine her passion for horseback riding with her desire to work with disabled youngsters to offer therapeutic horseback riding.

Jessica was fortunate in so many ways. She was bright and able to use her intellectual gifts to help her overcome her dyslexia. Her mother was a teacher who pursued specialized training so she could help Jessica and other dyslexic children master basic reading and spelling skills. Jessica was also fortunate that she qualified in third grade for public school learning disability support services; this support helped her acquire critical basic academic skills and relieved academic pressures through the implementation of educational modifications and accommodations, such as extended time. Even so, Jessica felt the pain of receiving poor grades, feeling dumb, and getting frustrated. However, with support at home and school, including excellent teaching, she was able to master basic skills, steadily build her confidence, learn to advocate for herself, and discover what she needed to do to succeed.

Not all dyslexic children are so fortunate. They may not have Jessica's intellectual gifts, or a mother committed to teaching and advocacy. They should, however, have teachers who advocate as best they can for appropriate, skilled instruction and critical educational accommodations and modifications. Parents and teachers must support the fragile self-esteem of these vulnerable children who need to learn that they, too, have strengths and talents that will help them meet the academic challenges they face and pursue their dreams.

# 10

# SUCCESS BEYOND WORDS

## Conclusion and Resources

## CONCLUSION

This book was written for all those seeking an accurate and current introduction to language-based reading and writing difficulties. The term *dyslexia* has now been defined by researchers in such a way that reliable identification of this condition is possible. Dyslexia can be distinguished from other kinds of reading and language difficulties that may arise from general cognitive disorders, other learning disorders, lack of opportunity to learn, or problems with comprehension that exist along with good word reading skills. Dyslexia affects individuals across a wide range of intellectual ability and at all socioeconomic levels. It is easiest to recognize in those who have notable talents and interests in areas other than reading and spelling, and who have high academic and career aspirations, but dyslexia is also common in average people who are working very hard to succeed in school and in life.

A unifying theme of this book is that dyslexia continues to affect individuals throughout life, even when their teachers and families have provided support, resources, and excellent instruction. To promote awareness of dyslexia at all stages of reading and academic development, we have described its manifestations from preschool to adulthood. Whether their reading, language, and writing problems are mild or severe, individuals with dyslexia face a series of challenges in school that change as they mature. Those challenges may affect life outside of and beyond school as well, including social interactions, recreational or athletic pursuits, choice of job or career, and management of daily tasks of living. Those with dyslexia deserve information, counseling, instruction, and accommodations throughout their academic careers even if they have overcome the most apparent difficulties with basic reading and writing skills.

The information provided in this book should help educators and families understand why we embrace the term *dyslexia*. True, the term is misunderstood by the public, many myths abound, and differentiating dyslexia from other kinds of learning problems is not always easy. It is true as well that the term is used for a wide range of conditions, from very mild problems to severe learning disorders. Nevertheless, something is lost with the more transparent term, *reading disability*. Dyslexia means *difficulty with words or language*, a term that encourages the user to associate a reading or spelling problem with the language processes that underlie it.

The term *dyslexia* also connotes the many scientific disciplines whose researchers have unraveled some of the mysteries of human language and literacy. Dyslexia is not a medical disorder, even though neurologists, geneticists, psychiatrists, neuro-psychologists, and other investigators trained in medical science have greatly enhanced our understanding of the nature of reading, writing, and language difficulty. Dyslexia remains a condition that requires educational intervention and treatment. Many programs, methods, and instructional techniques have proven value in helping students with dyslexia and related learning problems (see the resource list that follows).

Individuals with dyslexia face academic challenges that can be met with hard work, expert instruction, long-term planning, technology supports, and wise choices. They have succeeded in every profession, every vocation, and every academic discipline—even language-intensive fields such as medicine, law, and teaching. Some find their niches in less traditional lines of work such as deep sea fishing, customized automobile painting, golf course design or management, graphic arts, or the entertainment industry. Because they have had to cope with challenges every day, dyslexic individuals are often very resourceful and effective problem solvers, able to find ways around their challenges with spoken or written language. In other words, individuals with dyslexia often achieve successes in life in spite of their difficulties with words, through their resourcefulness, motivation, perseverance, and creativity.

# RESOURCES

## *Dyslexia, Learning Disabilities, and Attention Disorders*

### Attention Deficit Disorder Association (ADDA): *http://www.add.org*

ADDA provides information, resources, and networking to adults with AD/HD and to the professionals who work with them. The information and resources provided through the website focus on diagnoses, treatments, strategies, and techniques for helping adults with AD/HD lead better lives. Further, they offer an online directory for local support groups and for professionals who provide services for individuals with AD/HD.

### Children and Adults with Attention-Deficit / Hyperactivity Disorder (CHADD): *http://www.chadd.org/*

CHADD is composed of dedicated volunteers from around the country who play an integral part in the association's success by providing resources and encouragement to parents, educators, and professionals. They offer information about AD/HD, referrals, conferences, and training.

### Council for Learning Disabilities: *http://www.cldinternational.org/home.asp*

The Council for Learning Disabilities (CLD) is an international organization that promotes effective teaching and research. CLD is composed of professionals who represent diverse disciplines and who are committed to enhance the education and lifespan development of individuals with learning disabilities. The website features infosheets on various LD-related topics.

### International Dyslexia Association (IDA):
*http://www.interdys.org*

IDA is a nonprofit organization dedicated to helping individuals with dyslexia, their families, and the communities that support them. IDA is the oldest learning disabilities organization in the nation—providing the most comprehensive forum for parents, educators, and researchers to share their experiences, methods, and knowledge.

### Hello Friend: Ennis William Cosby Foundation:
*http://www.hellofriend.org*

This foundation equips teachers, parents, and students with the practical information and educational tools needed to understand and address the needs of all learners.

### Learning Disabilities Association of America (LDA):
*http://www.ldanatl.org/*

LDA offers specialized services designed to support and promote the success of individuals with learning disabilities across all aspects of life. The website features position papers and information about LD for parents, adults, teachers, professionals, publications, and research.

### LD OnLine: *http://www.ldonline.org/*

LD OnLine seeks to help children and adults reach their full potential by providing accurate and up-to-date information and advice about learning disabilities and AD/HD. The site features hundreds of helpful articles, monthly columns by noted experts, first person essays, children's writing and artwork, a comprehensive resource guide, a set of very active bulletin boards, and a referral directory of professionals, schools, and products.

## National Center for Learning Disabilities (NCLD): *http://www.ncld.org/*

NCLD provides essential information to parents, professionals, and individuals with learning disabilities, promotes research and programs to foster effective learning, and advocates for policies to protect and strengthen educational rights and opportunities.

## National Association for the Education of African American Children with Learning Disabilities: *http://www.aacld.org*

The National Association for the Education of African American Children with Learning Disabilities (NAEAACLD) links information and resources provided by an established network of individuals and organizations experienced in minority research and special education with parents, educators, and others responsible for providing an appropriate education for students, specifically African-American students.

## National Coalition on Auditory Processing Disorders, Inc.: *http://www.ncapd.org/php/*

The National Coalition on Auditory Processing Disorders, Inc. assists families and individuals affected by auditory processing disorders through education, support, and public awareness, as well as promoting auditory access of information for those affected by auditory processing disorders.

## National Dissemination Center for Children with Disabilities (NICHCY): *http://www.nichcy.org*

NICHCY is a central source of information on: disabilities in infants, toddlers, children, and youth; IDEA, which is the law authorizing special education; No Child Left Behind (as it relates to children with disabilities); and research-based information on effective educational practices.

### Reading Rockets: *http://www.readingrockets.org/*

Reading Rockets, a project of public television station WETA, aims to inform and inspire parents, teachers, childcare providers, administrators, and others who touch the life of a child by providing accurate, accessible information on how to teach kids to read and help those who struggle. They offer information on teaching strategies, publications, research and reports, and resources.

### Schwab Learning: *http://www.schwablearning.org*

Schwab Learning is a nonprofit organization dedicated to providing reliable, parent-friendly information from experts and parents. The extensive website offers information on LD, articles, publications, and a message board.

## *Multisensory Structured Language Education (MSLE)*

### Academic Language Therapy Association (ALTA): *http://www.altaread.org*

ALTA is an educational, structured, comprehensive, phonetic, multisensory approach for the remediation of dyslexia and/or written-language disorders. ALTA is a nonprofit national professional organization created for the purpose of establishing, maintaining, and promoting standards of education, practice, and professional conduct for Certified Academic Language Therapists. ALTA offers an online directory of therapists and a helpline for locating certified therapists.

### Academy of Orton-Gillingham Practitioners and Educators: *http://www.ortonacademy.org*

The Academy of Orton-Gillingham Practitioners and Educators (AOGPE) "certifies those individuals who have demonstrated competence as practitioners and educators of the Orton-Gillingham approach." Their website, an excellent resource for information about the Orton-Gillingham approach, provides information about the Academy, Orton and Gillingham, dyslexia, and training programs across the country.

### International Multisensory Structured Language Education Council (IMSLEC): *http://www.imslec.org/*

IMSLEC accredits quality Multisensory Structured Language Education (MSLE) training courses. These training programs offer extensive coursework and supervised teaching experience leading to professional certification. The training programs may be independent post-secondary training programs or may exist within already accredited institutions, such as colleges. The website includes a directory of IMSLEC accredited programs.

## *Accommodations and Technology*

### Alliance for Technology Access: *http://www.ataccess.org/*

The Alliance for Technology Access (ATA) is a national network of community-based resource centers, developers, vendors, and associates dedicated to providing information and support services to children and adults with disabilities, and increasing their use of standard, assistive, and information technologies. ATA's online resource area provides useful information about accessibility solutions, and ATA's local Resource Centers offer family members, educators, employers, legislators, and people with disabilities technical assistance and opportunities to explore computers, software, adaptive devices, and telecommunications systems.

### Benetech Bookshare: *http://bookshare.org*

Bookshare is a subscription-based service that gives print disabled people in the United States access to over 33,400 books and 150 national, regional, and local newspapers and magazines that are converted to Braille, large print, or text-to-speech audio files. Bookshare features the latest best sellers in fiction and nonfiction, computers and technology, sci-fi, romance, cooking, gardening, travel, children's titles, and K-12 and college-level textbooks.

### Center for Applied Special Technology (CAST): *http://www.cast.org/*

CAST's mission is to expand learning opportunities for all individuals, especially those with disabilities, through the research and development of innovative, technology-based educational resources and strategies. The website provides information on Universal Design for Learning (UDL), which is a framework for designing curricula that enable all individuals to gain knowledge, skills, and enthusiasm for learning. UDL provides rich supports for learning and reduces barriers to the curriculum while maintaining high achievement standards for all.

**Library Reproduction Service (LRS):**
*http://www.lrs-largeprint.com/contact.html*

LRS is a provider of large print reproductions to schools and other education providers across the United States and Canada.

**Recording for the Blind and Dyslexic (RFB&D):**
*http://www.rfbd.org*

RFB&D records educational and reference materials that are not available on tape or disc from other sources. RFB&D's library contains an extensive collection of audio-book titles in a broad variety of subjects, from literature and history to math and the sciences, at all academic levels, from kindergarten through post-graduate and professional. Anyone with a documented disability—including a visual impairment, learning disability, or other physical disability that makes reading standard print difficult or impossible—is eligible to use RFB&D's audio textbooks.

### *Advocacy and the IEP Process*

**Advocates for Justice and Education, Inc.:**
*http://www.aje-dc.org/*

This organization (local to D.C.) educates and trains parents, and those working with parents, about laws governing the education of children with disabilities or learning differences impeding their ability to learn and successfully matriculate through the public school system.

**The Council of Parent Attorneys and Advocates, Inc. (COPAA):** *http://www.copaa.org/news/idea04.html*

COPAA is an independent, nonprofit, tax-exempt organization of attorneys, advocates, and parents, whose primary mission is to secure high-quality educational services for children with disabilities. The organization does not provide direct services, individual advocacy, or representation to children with disabilities. Rather, COPAA's chief concern is that parents of children with disabilities have equal access to established legal protections by ensuring the availability and quality of legal and advocacy resources for parents of children with all types of disabilities. Through the website, parents can search the Attorney/Advocates database to find COPAA members in their area.

### Disability Rights Education and Defense Fund, Inc.: *http://www.dredf.org*

The Disability Rights Education and Defense Fund, Inc. (DREDF) is a national law and policy center dedicated to protecting and advancing the civil rights of people with disabilities through legislation, litigation, advocacy, technical assistance, and education. DREDF educates attorneys, advocates, persons with disabilities, and parents of children with disabilities about state and federal disability rights laws so they can use the laws as tools to challenge exclusion and discrimination, and advocate effectively for full participation in their communities.

### Families and Advocates Partnership for Education: *http://www.fape.org*

The Families and Advocates Partnership for Education (FAPE) project is a partnership that aims to improve the educational outcomes for children with disabilities. It links families, advocates, and self-advocates to information about the Individuals with Disabilities Education Act (IDEA).

### National Coalition for Parent Involvement in Education (NCPIE): *http://www.ncpie.org*

NCPIE advocates for the involvement of parents and families in their children's education, and fosters relationships between home, school, and community to enhance the education of the nation's young people. NCPIE serves as a clearinghouse for resources that help build and facilitate effective family-school partnerships.

### Parent Advocacy Coalition for Educational Rights (PACER): *http://www.pacer.org*

PACER Center expands opportunities and enhances the quality of life of children and young adults with disabilities and their families, based on the concept of parents helping parents. Staff is available to answer questions and offer one-on-one help.

### Parent Educational Advocacy Training Center (PEATC): *http://www.peatc.org/*

PEATC provides support, education, and training to families, schools, and professionals dedicated to helping children with LD. The website offers special education information, publications, and resource links.

### Parent Training and Information Centers and Community Parent Resource Centers: *http://www.taalliance.org/centers/*

Parent Training and Information Centers (PTIs) and Community Parent Resource Centers (CPRCs) in each state provide training and information to parents of infants, toddlers, children, and youth with disabilities and to professionals who work with children. They help families obtain appropriate education and services for their children with disabilities; work to improve educational results for all children; train and inform parents and professionals on a variety of topics; resolve problems between families and schools or other agencies; and connect children with disabilities to community resources that address their needs.

### Parents Engaged in Education Reform (PEER) Federation for Children with Special Needs: *http://www.fcsn.org/peer*

PEER is a national technical assistance project funded by the U.S. Department of Education, Office of Special Education Programs. PEER strives to increase the participation of parents of children with disabilities and their organizations in school reform efforts. The PEER Project provides opportunities for parents, parent organizations, and professionals to learn from each other about school restructuring efforts occurring in states and local communities.

### Technical Assistance Alliance for Parent Centers (TAAPC): *http://www.taalliance.org*

TAAPC supports a unified technical assistance system for the purpose of developing, assisting, and coordinating Parent Training and Information Projects and Community Parent Resource Centers under the Individuals with Disabilities Education Act (IDEA).

### Wrightslaw: *http://www.wrightslaw.com*

Wrightslaw provides parents, educators, advocates, and attorneys with accurate, reliable information about special education law, education law, and advocacy for children with disabilities. Wrightslaw offers thousands of articles, cases, and free resources about dozens of topics. Parents can learn how to build their team, get educated about their child's disability, find special education advocacy training, locate a parent group, and get legal and advocacy help.

## Private Schools

### National Association of Independent Schools (NAIS): *http://www.nais.org*

NAIS represents approximately 1,200 independent schools and associations in the United States and affiliates with independent schools abroad, as well. The website offers statistical data, resources, publications, conferences, information on financial aid, and a school search feature.

### National Association of Private Special Education Centers: *http://www.napsec.org/*

The National Association of Private Special Education Centers (NAPSEC) is a nonprofit association whose mission is to represent private special education centers and their leaders. NAPSEC promotes high-quality programs for individuals with disabilities and their families and advocates for access to the continuum of alternative placements and services.

## Higher Education

### Association on Higher Education and Disability (AHEAD): *http://www.ahead.org*

AHEAD is a professional association committed to full participation of persons with disabilities in postsecondary education, offering conferences, workshops, resources, and publications to higher education personnel. AHEAD members represent a diverse network of professionals who actively address disability issues on their campuses and in the field of higher education.

### CollegeView: *http://www.collegeview.com/*

CollegeView offers a searchable database of colleges intended to help students find the right college for their needs. Users can specify a search for colleges with programs for students with learning disabilities and many other parameters. The site also includes information on college applications, choosing a career, and financial aid.

### Council for Opportunity in Education (the Council): *http://www.coenet.us*

The Council advances and defends the ideal of equal educational opportunity in postsecondary education. The Council works in conjunction with colleges, universities, and agencies that host TRIO Programs to specifically help low-income and disabled Americans enter and graduate from college.

### Peterson's Guide: *http://www.petersons.com*

Peterson's Guide provides information about colleges and universities, career schools, graduate programs, distance learning, executive training, private secondary schools, summer opportunities, study abroad, financial aid, test preparation, and career exploration.

## Research and Reading Disabilities

### Florida Center for Reading and Research (FCRR): *http://www.fcrr.org/*

FCCR conducts extensive research on reading, reading growth, reading assessment, and reading instruction to contribute to the scientific knowledge of reading and benefit students in Florida and throughout the nation. Further, FCCR disseminates information about research-based practices related to literacy instruction and assessment for children in preschool through 12th grade.

### National Institute for Literacy: *http://www.nifl.gov/*

The National Institute for Literacy, a federal agency, provides leadership on literacy issues, including the improvement of reading instruction for children, youth, and adults. In consultation with the U.S. Departments of Education, Labor, and Health and Human Services, the Institute serves as a national resource on current, comprehensive literacy research, practice, and policy.

### National Research Center on Learning Disabilities: *http://www.nrcld.org/*

The National Research Center on Learning Disabilities (NRCLD) conducts research on the identification of learning disabilities; formulates implementation recommendations; disseminates findings; and provides technical assistance to national, state, and local constituencies.

### Vaughn Gross Center for Reading and Language Arts: *http://www.texasreading.org/utcrla/*

The Vaughn Gross Center for Reading and Language Arts,

located in the College of Education on the University of Texas at Austin campus, provides leadership to educators in effective reading instruction through its diversified research, technical assistance, and professional development projects. From translating research into practice to providing online professional development, the Center emphasizes scientifically based reading research and instruction. The Vaughn Gross Center seeks to improve reading instruction for all students, especially struggling readers, English language learners, and special education students.

### What Works Clearinghouse:
*http://www.whatworks.ed.gov/*

The What Works Clearinghouse (WWC) was established in 2002 by the U.S. Department of Education's Institute of Education Sciences to provide educators, policymakers, researchers, and the public with a central and trusted source of scientific evidence of what works in education. The WWC promotes informed education decision making through a set of easily accessible databases and user-friendly reports that provide education consumers with high-quality reviews of the effectiveness of replicable educational interventions (programs, products, practices, and policies) intended to improve student outcomes.

## *National Education Testing and Policy*

### National Center for Education Statistics (NCES, The Nation's Report Card):
*http://nces.ed.gov/nationsreportcard/*

NCES provides the only nationally representative and continuing assessment of what America's students know and can do in various subject areas, the National Assessment of Educational Progress (NAEP). NAEP does not provide scores for individual students or schools; instead, it offers results regarding subject-matter achievement, instructional experiences, and school environment for populations of students (e.g., fourth-graders) and groups within those populations (e.g., female students, Hispanic students). NAEP results are based on a sample of student populations of interest.

### Special Education Resources on the Internet (SERI): *http://www.seriweb.com*

SERI is a collection of links to Internet accessible information resources of interest to those involved in fields related to special education, which is designed to make online special education resources more easily and readily available in one location. SERI continually modifies, updates, and adds additional informative links.

### U.S. Department of Education: *http://www.ed.gov/*

The U.S. Department of Education (ED) is the agency of the federal government that establishes policy for, administers, and coordinates most federal assistance to education. The ED website offers resources and information for students, parents, teachers, and administrators.

### IDEA Partnership: *http://www.ideapartnership.org*

The IDEA Partnership reflects the collaborative work of more than 55 national organizations, technical assistance providers, and organizations and agencies at state and local levels. The website offers extensive resources on a variety of topics and related issues regarding the implementation of NCLB, IDEA, and other legislation. Together with the Office of Special Education Programs (OSEP), the Partner Organizations form a community that is dedicated to improving outcomes for students and youth with disabilities by joining state agencies and stakeholders through shared work and learning.

## Professional Organizations

### American Academy of Child and Adolescent Psychiatry: *http://www.aacap.org*

The American Academy of Child and Adolescent Psychiatry (AACAP) is a national professional medical association dedicated to treating and improving the quality of life for children, adolescents, and families. This site provides information about ADD, AD/HD, and other issues that affect children, teenagers, and their families. The AACAP website offers information on when and where parents can seek help for their children and includes a search tool for finding child and adolescent psychiatrists in their area.

### Association of Educational Therapists: *http://www.aetonline.org*

The Association of Educational Therapists (AET) is a national professional association for educational therapists. Educational therapists provide a broad range of individualized educational interventions for children and adults with learning disabilities and other learning challenges. The website features a parent's guide to educational therapy and provides information about standards for the professional practice of educational therapy and professional development opportunities.

### Academic Language Therapy Association (ALTA): *http://www.altaread.org*

ALTA is an educational, structured, comprehensive, phonetic, multisensory approach for the remediation of dyslexia and/or written-language disorders. ALTA is a nonprofit national professional organization created for the purpose of establishing, maintaining, and promoting standards of education, practice, and professional conduct for Certified Academic Language Therapists. ALTA offers an online directory of therapists and a helpline for locating certified therapists.

### Academy of Orton-Gillingham Practitioners and Educators: *http://www.ortonacademy.org*

The Academy of Orton-Gillingham Practitioners and Educators (AOGPE) "certifies those individuals who have demonstrated competence as practitioners and educators of the Orton-Gillingham approach." Their website, an excellent resource for information about the Orton-Gillingham approach, provides information about the Academy, Orton and Gillingham, dyslexia, and training programs across the country.

### American Speech-Language-Hearing Association (ASHA): *http://www.asha.org*

ASHA is the professional, scientific, and credentialing association for audiologists; speech-language pathologists; and speech, language, and hearing scientists. ASHA offers an online directory of audiology and speech-language pathology programs and private practitioners for individuals who want to find qualified audiologists and speech-language pathologists.

### Council for Exceptional Children (CEC):
*http://www.cec.sped.org/*

CEC provides information to teachers and other service providers about special education issues for students with disabilities and/or gifted students. CEC's Division for Learning Disabilities (DLD) provides information and resources for teaching students with learning disabilities through its website, TeachingLD (*http://www.teachingld. org*). In addition to serving as a resource for members of DLD, TeachingLD.org publishes content about assessment, instruction, and policy related to learning disabilities. Readers can find information about curriculum-based measurement (CBM) for monitoring student progress; teaching methods, such as co-teaching and direct instruction; and current issues such as response-to-intervention (RTI) models.

### National Association of School Psychologists (NASP)
*http://www.nasponline.org/*

The National Association of School Psychologists (NASP) is a not-for-profit association representing school psychologists from across the United States and other countries. The NASP website provides information designed to support efforts to enhance the mental health and educational competence of all children. The website is also a useful resource for members, parents, educators, and others interested in helping children and their families. NASP publishes summaries of research on issues such as grade retention, testing, disciplinary practices, and management of exceptional children.

**National Association of State Directors of Special Education (NASDSE):** *http://nasdse.org/*

NASDSE is a services-focused organization to help state education agencies promote and support specially designed instruction and related services for children and youth with disabilities to maximize educational outcomes.

# References

## Chapter 1: What Is Dyslexia?

Brady, S. A., & Shankweiler, D. P. (Eds.). (1991). *Phonological processes in literacy*. Hillsdale, NJ: Erlbaum.

Ehri, L., & Snowling, M. (2004). Developmental variation in word recognition. In A. C. Stone, E. R. Silliman, B. J. Ehren, & K. Apel (Eds.), *Handbook of language and literacy: Development and disorders* (pp. 443–460). New York: Guilford Press.

Fletcher, J. M., Morris, R. D., & Lyon, G. R. (2003). Classification and definition of learning disabilities: An integrative perspective. In H. L. Swanson, K. R. Harris, & S. Graham (Eds.), *Handbook of learning disabilities* (pp. 30–56). New York: Guilford Publications.

Francis, D. J., Shaywitz, S. E., Stuebing, K. K., Shaywitz, B. A., & Fletcher, J. M. (1996). Developmental lag versus deficit models of reading disability: A longitudinal, individual growth curves analysis. *Journal of Educational Psychology, 88*, 3–17.

Joshi, M., & Aaron, P. G. (2000). The component model of reading: Simple view of reading made a little more complex. *Reading Psychology, 21*, 85–87.

Liberman, I. Y., & Shankweiler, D. (1985). Phonology and the problems of learning to read and write. *Remedial and Special Education, 6*, 8–17.

Lyon, G. R., Fletcher, J. M., Shaywitz, S. E., Shaywitz, B. A., Torgesen, J. K., Wood, F. B., et al. (2001). Rethinking learning disabilities. In C. E. Finn, Jr., A. J. Rotherham, & C. R. Hokanson, Jr. (Eds.), *Rethinking special education for a new century* (pp. 259–287). Washington, DC: Thomas B. Fordham Foundation and Progressive Policy Institute.

Lyon, G. R., Shaywitz, S. E., & Shaywitz, B. A. (2003). A definition of dyslexia. *Annals of Dyslexia, 53,* 1–14.

McCardle, P., & Chhabra, V. (2004). *The voice of evidence in reading research.* Baltimore: Paul Brookes.

Share, D., & Stanovich, K. (1995). Cognitive processes in early reading development: Accommodating individual differences into a model of acquisition. *Issues in Education: Contributions to Educational Psychology, 1,* 1–57.

Shaywitz, S. E. (2003). *Overcoming dyslexia: A new and complete science-based program for reading problems at any level.* New York: Knopf.

Shaywitz, S. E., Fletcher, J. M., Holahan, J. M., Schneider, A. E., Marchione, K. E., Stuebing, K. K., et al. (1999). Persistence of dyslexia: The Connecticut longitudinal study at adolescence. *Pediatrics, 104,* 1351–1359.

Vellutino, F. R., Fletcher, J. M., Scanlon, D. M., & Snowling, M. J. (2004). Specific reading disability (dyslexia): What have we learned in the past four decades? *Journal of Child Psychiatry and Psychology, 45,* 2–40.

Wolf, M., & Bowers, P. G. (1999). The double deficit hypothesis for the developmental dyslexias. *Journal of Educational Psychology, 91,* 415–438.

## Chapter 2: Dyslexia: Manifestations from Preschool to Adulthood

Adams, M., Foorman, B. R., Lundberg, I., & Beeler, T. (1998). The elusive phoneme. *American Educator, 22*(1&2), 18–22.

Cunningham, A., & Stanovich, K. (1991). Tracking the unique effects of print exposure in children: Associations with vocabulary, general knowledge, and spelling. *Journal of Educational Psychology, 83*(2), 264–274.

Hasbrouck, J. E., & Tindal, J. (2005). *Oral Reading Fluency: 90 Years of Assessment* (BRT Tech. Rep. No. 33). Eugene, OR: Behavioral Research and Teaching.

Lonigan, C. J. (2003). Development and promotion of emergent literacy skills in children at-risk of reading difficulties. In B. R. Foorman (Ed.), *Preventing and remediating reading difficulties* (pp. 23–50). Timonium, MD: York Press.

Treiman, R., & Bourassa, D. (2000). The development of spelling skill. *Topics in Language Disorders, 20*(3), 1–18.

## Chapter 3: How Common Is the Problem?

Hoskyn, M., & Swanson, H. L. (2000). Cognitive processing of low achievers and children with reading disabilities: A selective meta-analytic review of the published literature. *The School Psychology Review, 29,* 102–119.

National Center for Educational Statistics (NCES) (2005). *National Assessment of Educational Progress: The Nation's Report Card.* Washington, DC: U.S. Department of Education.

President's Commission on Excellence in Special Education (2002). *A new era: Revitalizing special education for children and their families.* Washington, DC: U.S. Department of Education.

Stanovich, K. (1993). The construct validity of discrepancy definition of reading disabilities. In G. R. Lyon, D. B. Gray, J. F. Kavanagh, & N. A. Krasnegor (Eds.), *Better understanding learning disabilities: New views from research and their implications for education and public policies* (pp. 273–307). Baltimore: Paul H. Brookes.

Stuebing, K. K., Fletcher, J. M., LeDoux, J. M., Lyon, G. R., Shaywitz, S. E., & Shaywitz, B. A. (2002). Validity of IQ-discrepancy classifications of reading disabilities: A meta-analysis. *American Educational Research Journal, 39,* 469–518.

## Chapter 4: Identifying the Child at Risk

Berninger, V., & Amtmann, D. (2003). Preventing written expression disabilities through early and continuing assessment and intervention for handwriting and/or spelling problems: Research into practice. In H. L. Swanson, K. R. Harris, & S. Graham (Eds.), *Handbook of learning disabilities* (pp. 345–363). New York: Guilford Press.

Fuchs, D., Mock, D., Morgan, P., & Young, C. (2003). Responsiveness-to-intervention: Definitions, evidence, and implications for the learning disabilities construct. *Learning Disabilities Research and Practice, 18,* 157–171.

Good, R. H., Simmons, D. C., & Kameenui, E. (2001). The importance and decision-making utility of a continuum of fluency-based indicators of foundational reading skills for third-grade high-stakes outcomes. *Scientific Studies of Reading, 5,* 257–288.

Gresham, F. M. (2002). Responsiveness to intervention: An alternative approach to the identification of learning disabilities. In R. Bradley, L. Danielson, & D. P. Hallahan (Eds.), *Identification of learning disabilities: Research to practice* (pp. 467–564). Mahwah, NJ: Erlbaum.

Schatschneider, C., & Torgesen, J. K. (2004). Using our current understanding of dyslexia to support early identification and intervention. *Journal of Child Neurology, 19*(10), 759–765.

Shinn, M. R. (1998). *Advanced applications of curriculum-based measurement.* New York, NY: Guilford Press.

Torgesen, J. K. (2004). Preventing early reading failure—and its devastating downward spiral: The evidence for early intervention. *American Educator, 28*(3), 6–19, 45–47.

Vaughn, S., & Fuchs, L. S. (2003). Redefining learning disabilities as inadequate response to instruction: The promise and potential problems. *Learning Disabilities Research & Practice, 18*, 137–146.

## Chapter 5: Genetics, the Brain, and Dyslexia

Eden, G. & Moats, L. (2002). The role of neuroscience in the remediation of students with dyslexia. *Nature Neuroscience, 5*, 1080–1084.

Gayan, J., & Olson, R. K. (2003). Genetic and environmental influences on individual differences in printed word recognition. *Journal of Experimental Child Psychology, 84*, 97–123.

Gilger, J. W., & Wise, S. E. (2004). Genetic correlates of language and literacy impairments. In C. A. Stone, E. R. Silliman, B. J. Ehren, & K. Apel (Eds.), *Handbook of language and literacy: Development and disorders* (pp. 25–48). New York: Guilford.

Mody, M. (2004). Neurobiological correlates of language and reading impairments. In C. A. Stone, E. R. Silliman, B. J. Ehren, & K. Apel (Eds.), *Handbook of language and literacy: Development and disorders* (pp. 49–72). New York: Guilford.

Olson, R. K. (2004). SSSR, environment, and genes. *Scientific Studies of Reading, 8*(2), 111–124.

Simos, P. G., Fletcher, J. M., Bergman, E., Breier, J. I., Foorman, B. R., Castillo, E. M., et al. (2002). Dyslexia-specific brain activation profile becomes normal following successful remedial training. *Neurology, 58*, 1203–1213.

## Chapter 6: Expert Teaching Is the Treatment

Armbruster, B., Lehr, F., & Osborn, J. (2001). *Put reading first: The research building blocks for teaching children to read, kindergarten through grade 3.* Washington, DC: National Institute for Literacy.

Biemiller, A. (1999). *Language and reading success.* Cambridge, MA: Brookline Books.

Blachman, B. A., Ball, E. W., Black, R. S., & Tangel, D. M. (1994). Kindergarten teachers develop phoneme awareness in low-income, inner-city classrooms: Does it make a difference? *Reading and Writing: An Interdisciplinary Journal, 6,* 1–18.

Blachman, B. A., Schatschneider, C., Fletcher, J. M., Francis, D. J., Clonan, S., Shaywitz, B., & Shaywitz, S. (2004). Effects of intensive reading remediation for second and third graders. *Journal of Educational Psychology, 96,* 444–461.

Carlisle, J., & Rice, M. S. (2003). *Reading comprehension: Research-based principles and practices.* Timonium, MD: York Press.

Christenson, C. A., & Bowey, J. A. (2005). The efficacy of orthographic rime, grapheme-phoneme correspondence, and implicit phonics approaches to teaching decoding skills. *Scientific Studies of Reading, 9*(4), 327–349.

Coyne, M. D., Kame'enui, E. J., Simmons, D. C., & Harn, B. A. (2004). Beginning reading intervention as inoculation or insulin: First-grade reading performance of strong responders to kindergarten intervention. *Journal of Learning Disabilities, 37,* 90–104.

Denton, C., Foorman, B. R., & Mathes, G. G. (2003). Schools that "Beat the Odds"—Implications for reading instruction. *Remedial and Special Education, 24,* 258–261.

Fletcher, J. M., Lyon, G. R., Fuchs, L. S., Barnes, M. A. (2007). *Learning disabilities: From identification to intervention.* New York: Guilford.

Foorman, B. R., Francis, D. J., Fletcher, J. M., Schatschneider, C., & Mehta, P. (1998). The role of instruction in learning to read: Preventing reading failure in at-risk-children. *Journal of Educational Psychology, 90,* 37–55.

Foorman, B. R., & Moats, L. C. (2004). Conditions for sustaining research-based practices in early reading instruction. *Remedial and Special Education, 25*(1), 51–60.

Fuchs, L., & Fuchs, D. (1999). Monitoring student progress toward the development of reading competence: A review of three forms of classroom-based assessment. *The School Psychology Review, 28,* 659–671.

Hasbrouck, J., & Tindal, G. A. (2006). Oral reading fluency norms: A valuable assessment tool for reading teachers. *The Reading Teacher, 59*(7), 636–644.

Jetton, T. L., and Dole, J. A. (Eds.). (2004). *Adolescent literacy research and practice.* New York: Guilford.

Kuhn, M. R., & Stahl, S. A. (2003). Fluency: A review of developmental and remedial practices. *Journal of Educational Psychology, 95,* 3–21.

Mathes, P. G., Denton, C. A., Fletcher, J. M., Anthony, J. L., Francis, D. J., & Schatschneider, C. (2005). An evaluation of two reading interventions derived from diverse models. *Reading Research Quarterly, 40,* 148–182.

National Institutes of Child Health and Human Development (NICHD). (2000). *Report of the National Reading Panel: Teaching children to read—An evidence-based assessment of the scientific research literature on reading and its implications for reading instruction.* Bethesda, MD: NICHD, NIH. Retrieved August 21, 2007, from http://www.nationalreadingpanel.org/default.htm

Rayner, K., Foorman, B. F., Perfetti, C. A., Pesetsky, D., & Seidenberg, M. S. (2001). How psychological science informs the teaching of reading. *Psychological Science in the Public Interest, 2*(2), 31–74.

Seabaugh, G. O., & Schumaker, J. B. (1993). The effects of self-regulation training on the academic productivity of secondary students with learning problems. *Journal of Behavioral Education, 4*, 109–133.

Schumaker, J. B., Deshler, D. D., & McKnight, P. (2002). Ensuring success in the secondary general education curriculum through the use of teaching routines. In M. A. Shinn, H. M. Walker, & G. Stoner (Eds.), *Interventions for academic and behavior problems II: Preventive and remedial approaches* (pp. 791–823). Bethesda, MD: NASP Publications.

Tangel, D. M., & Blachman, B. A. (1995). Effect of phoneme awareness instruction on the invented spelling of first-grade children: A one-year follow-up. *Journal of Reading Behavior, 27*, 153–185.

## Chapter 7: Severe Dyslexia and Other Learning Disabilities

Alexander, A., & Slinger-Constant, A. (2004). Current status of treatments for dyslexia: Critical review. *Journal of Child Neurology, 19*(10), 744–758.

Berninger, V., & Richards, T. (2002). *Brain literacy for educators and psychologists.* Amsterdam: Academic Press.

Birsh, J. (2005). *Multisensory teaching of basic language skills* (2nd ed.). Baltimore: Paul H. Brookes.

Denton, C. A., & Mathes, P. G. (2003). Intervention for struggling readers: Possibilities and challenges. In B. R. Foorman (Ed.), *Preventing and remediating reading difficulties* (pp. 229–252). Timonium, MD: York Press.

Graham, S., & Harris, K. R. (2003). Students with learning disabilities and the process of writing: A meta-analysis of SRSD studies. In H. L. Swanson, K. R. Harris, & S. Graham (Eds.), *Handbook of learning disabilities* (pp. 323–344). New York: Guilford Press.

Lovett, M. W., Lacerenza, L., Borden, S. L., Frijters, J. C., Steinbach, K. A., & DePalma, M. (2000). Components of effective remediation for developmental reading disabilities: Combining phonological and strategy-based instruction to improve outcomes. *Journal of Educational Psychology, 92,* 263–283.

Lovett, M. W., Lacerenza, L., Murphy, D., Steinbach, K. A., DePalma, M., & Frijters, J. C. (2005). The importance of multi-component interventions for children and adolescents who are struggling readers. In S. O. Richardson, & J. Gilger (Eds.), *Research-based education and intervention: What we need to know* (pp. 67–102). Baltimore: International Dyslexia Association.

Olson, R. K. (2006). Genes, environment, and dyslexia: The 2005 Norman Geschwind Memorial Lecture. *Annals of Dyslexia, 56*(2), 205–238.

Shaywitz, S. E. (2003). *Overcoming dyslexia: A new and complete science-based program for reading problems at any level.* New York: Knopf.

Swanson, H. L., Hoskyn, M., & Lee, C. (1999). *Interventions for students with learning disabilities: A meta-analysis of treatment outcome.* New York: Guilford.

Torgesen, J. K. (2005). Remedial interventions for students with dyslexia: National goals and current accomplishments. In S. O. Richardson, & J. Gilger (Eds.), *Research-based education and intervention: What we need to know* (pp. 103–123). Baltimore: International Dyslexia Association.

Torgesen, J. K., Alexander, A. W., Wagner, R. K., Rashotte, C. A., Voeller, K. K. S., & Conway, T. (2001). Intensive remedial instruction for children with severe reading disabilities: Immediate and long-term outcomes from two instructional approaches. *Journal of Learning Disabilities, 34*, 33–58.

Vellutino, F. R., & Scanlon, D. M. (2002). The interactive strategies approach to reading intervention. *Contemporary Educational Psychology, 27*, 573–635.

## Chapter 8: Emotional Consequences of Dyslexia and Other Reading Problems

Huntington, D., & Bender, W. (1993). Adolescents with learning disabilities at risk: Emotional well-being, depression, and suicide. *Journal of Learning Disabilities, 26*, 159–166.

Olson, R. K. (2006). Genes, environment, and dyslexia: The 2005 Norman Geschwind Memorial Lecture. *Annals of Dyslexia, 56*(2), 205–238.

Ryan, M. (2000). *The other sixteen hours: The social and emotional problems of dyslexia* (Orton Emeritus Series). Baltimore: The International Dyslexia Association.

Spekman, N., Goldberg, R., & Herman, K. (1993). An exploration of risk and resilience in the lives of individuals with learning disabilities. *Learning Disabilities Research and Practice, 8*, 11–18.

# Index

Page references followed by *t* and f indicate tables and figures, respectively.